PALEO DIET
FOR WEIGHT LOSS

Author

Barbara E. Martin

Contents

People who make the switch to the paleo diet are always amazed by how much it boosts their energy and mood, improves their health and vitality, and makes them feel great every day. But despite these amazing health benefits, many people find that even after adopting a paleo diet, they're still struggling to lose weight!

Luckily, it doesn't have to be this way. With the right know-how, you can make some easy tweaks to the paleo diet that will crank up the fat-burning potential of the diet and allow you to melt pounds away faster than you ever thought possible.

In *Paleo for Weight Loss*, you'll learn dozens of delicious paleo recipes specifically designed for weight loss on the paleo diet. Each recipe is strategically targeted to be low in carbohydrates, fully compliant with paleo principles, rich in nutrients, and best of all, absolutely delicious!

Some of these delicious fat-burning recipes include:

- Lamb and Bacon Meatballs

- Thai Coconut Shrimp Soup

- Spicy Bison Burgers

- Pesto Scrambled Eggs

- Chipotle Lime Salmon

- Paleo Mocha Brownies

...and many more!

All the recipes in *Paleo for Weight Loss* are low carb, paleo/primal friendly, completely free from grains, gluten, soy, legumes, and refined sugars, and made with real, whole foods. Even better, they're also easy to make, require no special equipment, and are absolutely delicious!

So without further ado, let's get started!

One of the great things about the paleo diet is that even though it's primarily designed to improve your health (and all the related benefits like increased longevity, energy, disease resistance, and mental focus), it's also great for losing weight. In fact, many people who adopt the paleo diet for health reasons find that they lose weight without even trying! This is a natural side effect of eating a diet that is A) extremely nutrient-rich, B) low in carbs and high in protein and healthy fats, and C) based around nourishing, satisfying whole foods.

This is why, if one of your goals is to lose weight, we recommend that you start by just following a basic, healthy paleo diet, without focusing on weight loss at first. This allows you to get comfortable with the basics of the paleo diet (which can often be tricky at first, because it's a big lifestyle shift for many people), and make your transition to paleo as easy as possible without worrying about weight loss. Not only will this make the transition to paleo easier and more enjoyable, but as a bonus, most people will find that consistently eating paleo causes them to naturally shed unwanted bodyfat without even trying.

Once you're comfortable with the basics of the paleo diet, however, you may find that you aren't losing weight as fast as you want, or even at all! This is totally normal; just because you're eating healthy food doesn't mean you'll lose weight. Healthy eating habits will tend to reduce your appetite, as well as creating an ideal environment for fat loss in your body by optimizing your hormones, metabolism, calorie partitioning, and a host of other factors. However, you're still perfectly capable of eating surplus calories, and even if those calories are coming from healthy foods, a large enough surplus will still lead to weight gain!

The paleo diet in and of itself isn't a weight loss diet, so if losing weight is something you routinely struggle with, you may need to adopt some specific strategies along with the basic principles of healthy paleo eating in order to effectively burn off that unwanted bodyfat.

Remember that getting comfortable with paleo, and fully making the transition to eating paleo on a very consistent basis, is critically important as a starting point – be sure to focus on this basic lifestyle transition exclusively for the first few months of your paleo journey, and you'll make things way easier on yourself once the basic habits of paleo eating have already become second-nature to you.

Once you've reached the point where eating paleo is comfortable for you, and you'd like to start focusing more on losing weight, there are a few simple strategies that you can implement (in conjunction with the basic principles of the paleo diet) to optimize the paleo diet for fat loss. We'll discuss a few supplementary strategies later in this chapter, but when it comes to weight loss, the paleo diet mostly focuses on one simple strategy: reducing your consumption of carbohydrates.

The Benefits of Cutting Carbs for Weight Loss

As you know by now, the paleo diet is much more than just a "low carb diet"; in fact, depending on your personal preferences, food tolerances, and physical activity level, paleo doesn't necessarily need to be particularly low carb at all. But reducing carbohydrate consumption is considered by many followers of the paleo diet to not only be optimal for health, but also the most effective way to lose weight.

Reducing the amount of carbohydrates you consume (and by the same token, replacing them with protein and healthy fats), has a number of positive effects that stack up to create a powerful fat burning environment in your body. Reducing your carb intake will reduce the spikes in blood sugar and insulin that promote fat storage, increase your body's insulin sensitivity, reduce appetite (which leads to a natural reduction in your calorie intake), and will overall just switch your body into "fat burning mode".

As an added benefit, eating a low carb paleo diet will typically allow you to lose weight without counting calories! You don't need to weigh or measure your food, or keep a food journal; the absolute most you'll have to do is keep a rough estimate of how many grams of carbohydrate you're eating in a given day, and even this extra step is usually unnecessary. All you really need to do is focus on eating foods from the lower-carb spectrum of the paleo diet, like meat, eggs, and vegetables (as well as the accompanying herbs and spices that make them delicious!), and if you base most of your meals around these foods, there's a good chance you'll be able to lose weight without counting, measuring, or recording a single calorie!

So with all these benefits in mind, exactly how much should you be cutting carbs in order to lose weight as quickly, efficiently, and easily as possible?

Determining Your Ideal Carb Intake

There are a number of factors to consider when determining how many carbs you should be eating in a given day for achieving the optimal balance between weight loss and simple ease and convenience. We're going to give you some specific targets in a second, but before you decide exactly what your personal intake should be, there are a few guidelines you should keep in mind:

Measuring carbs

The carbohydrate targets listed below are, of course, quantified using numbers; specifically, how many grams of carbohydrate per day you should be eating for a specific goal. This doesn't necessarily mean that you need to literally keep a running tally of your daily carb intake in order to lose weight.

You certainly *can* track your carbs if you find that it helps you stay on track, but most people can get by without doing this. When you're first getting started, you'll probably need to look up the amount of carbs found in various paleo food groups you eat frequently (fruit, nuts, seeds, sweet potatoes, honey, etc). But once you get a solid picture of which foods are high-carb, moderate-carb, and low-carb, most paleo dieters find that they don't need to actually keep track in order to cut their carbs to approximately the right level for their goals.

Basically, our goal with the numerical guidelines listed below is just to give you an objective starting point to begin experimenting.

Adjusting for your activity level

In general, the more physically active you are, the more carbs you can eat while still losing weight. In fact, the majority of athletic, very physically active people find that if they let their carb intake dip too low, their mood, energy levels, and even athletic performance actually gets worse! So if you don't work out very often, you should probably be on the lower end of the spectrum, but if you're very physically active, you can experiment with slightly higher carb intakes and see how it affects your weight loss.

Adjusting for your personal physiology

First and most obviously, the following guidelines for carb intake are somewhat relative, and are geared towards an "average" person. However, it goes without saying that a six foot tall man is going to consume a different amount of food than a five foot tall woman, and therefore these two people are also going to consume different amounts of carbs. In this example, the large man's "fat burning zone" may be anything under 150 grams of carbs per day, while the petite woman's zone may be anything under 100 grams per day. So remember to adjust the numbers listed below to account for your body size if necessary.

In addition to this, there are many people who report anecdotally that they just *feel* better eating higher or lower amounts of carbs. On one end of the spectrum, some people find that their energy levels and mental focus are best when they keep their carb intake super low, while some people find that if they cut carbs too much they feel groggy and tired all the time. These reports are anecdotal, and technically don't have anything to do directly with weight loss, however they illustrate an important principle: if you find that eating within a certain carb range makes you feel better, listen to your body! The main point of living the paleo lifestyle is to feel great, not lousy. Plus, feeling lousy is going to prevent you from losing weight anyway, since it will make your diet unsustainable.

The takeaway from this is that if you start cutting carbs a bit aggressively in order to lose weight as quickly as possible, but you feel bad as a result, don't be afraid to scale it back a bit and reintroduce a few carbs to your diet. Slow and steady wins the race, and you're going to want to enjoy the benefits of eating a healthy paleo diet for the rest of your life; so make sure you're able to enjoy it!

Is it safe / healthy to cut carbs?

It should be noted that, although your body absolutely needs protein and fat in order to function (you literally cannot survive without them), it doesn't really need carbohydrates. In practice, carbs are useful and beneficial, because they allow you to have a more diverse, interesting diet, an easy way to get more nutrients (via fruit, nuts, seeds, etc), and make many people feel more energetic, particularly if they're physically active.

However, purely from a health standpoint, carbs aren't technically necessary to include in your diet, which means that you don't have to worry about a low carb diet being bad for your health. As long as you're getting enough nutrients from other sources (like veggies, pastured eggs, and organ meats), you can eat as few carbs as you want.

Please note that if you have any medical conditions that influence your blood sugar, insulin, or other factors related to consuming carbohydrates (most notably diabetes), or if you're taking any medication that might affect how your body responds to carbohydrates, you should carefully consult with your doctor before drastically changing your carb intake. The paleo diet is very healthy and safe, and in fact, many people even use it to manage chronic conditions like diabetes. But if you have a serious health condition, it's always best to play it safe!

Carb Intake Guidelines

With the above criteria in mind, here are some general guidelines for how many grams of carbohydrate you should be eating per day in order to achieve various levels of weight loss or weight maintenance. The guidelines are organized into rough "levels" of carb intake (each one spanning a small range to accommodate individual differences), and a description of how each level can potentially fit your personal situation and goals.

300+ grams/day

The amount eaten by the average person on the "Standard American Diet", and a fairly normal level to reach if you're scarfing down bread and sugar with every meal. A bit harder to reach with a paleo diet, unless you're eating a pretty large amount of honey, fruit, and/or sweet potatoes, as well as packing away quite a bit of total food. Almost certainly unhealthy, and definitely not conducive to weight loss, unless you're a very active athlete.

200-300 grams/day

Probably the upper limit of "safe" for the paleo diet, and only if you're very physically active. For active or particularly large individuals, this level might be doable for weight maintenance, as long as all the carbs are coming from paleo foods. Even then, this level of carb intake will almost never result in weight loss, unless you're very physically active, or using other strategies like calorie-counting. The average person, even eating an otherwise healthy paleo diet, will probably see slow, steady weight gain at this level. Not necessarily recommended for the goals of the average person, but a possible "zone" for active and larger people (particularly towards the bottom of the spectrum).

150-200 grams/day

In practice, for the average person this will be the upper limit of carb intake that will still allow for weigh maintenance. Maintaining weight in this range will probably still require moderate amounts of physical activity (unless you're fairly large), and very few people will experience actual weight loss in this range (unless you have a fairly high amount of excess bodyfat). For many (but by no means all) people, staying moderately active and eating a healthy paleo diet will allow them to comfortably stay at this level while maintaining a healthy weight.

100-150 grams/day

The beginning of the "fat burning zone" for the vast majority of people, preferably in conjunction with some physical activity. Possibly not enough for very active individuals to achieve their best athletic performance, but still fine for most activity levels. For the average person looking to lose weight, this is an ideal starting point for slowly, gradually, and easily burning fat over time, without the need for other strategies like calorie-counting or large amounts of exercise.

Since this level of intake is pretty moderate, eating habits and carb intake need to also be pretty consistent in order to maintain this weight loss over the long term. However, consistency is relatively easy at this level, since it still allows for moderate consumption of fruit, starchy root vegetables (like sweet potatoes), and paleo sweeteners (like honey). Lastly, for people who are particularly prone to gain weight, fairly inactive, smaller in stature, or who just want to maintain a very low bodyfat percentage, this might be more of a weight-maintenance level.

50-100 grams/day

The beginning of accelerated fat loss for most people. Heavier people will see relatively fast weight loss at this level, particularly in the first few weeks (after which weight loss will slow down but still continue at a steady rate). Most people who are already at a healthy starting weight will also be able to use this level of intake to get down to lower bodyfat percentages if desired. Most people will experience some degree of *ketosis* (burning extra fat to create *ketones*, which fill in where the body would normally burn glucose).

This level is not recommended as a long-term level of carb intake for most people, since diet becomes somewhat restrictive at this point, allowing mostly for intake of relatively small amounts of fruit with little or no sweeteners. Some people may also experience a reduction in energy levels at this level, possibly since calorie intake will naturally go down fairly significantly.

More vegetables and nutrient-rich animal foods (like organ meats and pastured eggs) should be eaten at this level, to keep nutrient intake high in the absence of a more diverse diet. After eating at this level for several months and losing a good amount of weight, most people will want to bump up their carb intake to a slightly higher level for maintenance purposes. This is rarely a good zone for very active people to be in, but occasionally useful for people who are inactive, suffering from blood sugar issues like pre-diabetes, or who simply feel subjectively "better" when reducing carbs in their diet (particularly sugars).

0-50 grams/day

Sharply accelerated fat loss for anyone in any situation, including a definite state of ketosis. It's almost impossible to overeat at this level, and in fact many people will need to be careful not to eat *too little* (since reducing calorie intake too sharply can sometimes lead to hunger cravings and reduced energy levels if you're not careful).

Most carbs at this level are coming from vegetables, with some nuts, nut butters, coconut products and miscellaneous items contributing the few remaining carbs; in all likelihood, no fruit, starches, or sweeteners are eaten at this level. Increasing consumption of vegetables, pastured eggs, and organ meats is vital to ensure proper nutrient intake, and if these foods can't be eaten regularly supplementation is a good idea.

Even the smallest, least active person will be able to lose weigh at this level, as well as people looking to reach very low bodyfat percentages. However, compliance becomes tricky, since the diet is now very restrictive. Definitely not recommended for long-term use; this level of intake can be used for rapid weight loss, or to get some medical conditions like pre-diabetes under control, before returning to higher levels of carb intake for weight maintenance. Highly effective for weight loss, but requires discipline to implement consistently.

Optimizing and Troubleshooting

Although weight loss with the paleo diet is usually relatively simple, there are a lot of little ways that people can accidentally slow their progress down, or even cause weight loss to stall entirely. By the same token, there are a number of small tips, tricks, and refinements to the basic paleo weight loss template that can help speed up or optimize the process of losing weight. We're going to discuss both of these types of strategies here, since many of these strategies can go either way: if not implemented properly they can slow your weight loss down, and if implemented well they can speed it up.

Keep in mind that it's normal for weight loss to slow down or even *temporarily* plateau after some initial success. This an inescapable part of the process, and perfectly healthy, so don't get discouraged and give up if you've had trouble losing weight with paleo, or if you aren't losing it as fast as you'd like. Instead of giving up altogether, try using some of the tips below and see if they speed things up for you.

Eat more protein vs. fat

The primary method for weight loss that the paleo diet focuses on is reducing carb intake, and once carbs are cut the protein and fat usually take care of themselves. However, it can also be extremely helpful for weight loss purposes to not only *decrease* carb intake, but also to *increase* protein intake. In fact, some experts believe that the main reason why low-carb diets work is because they usually result in an automatic increase in protein intake (since protein and fat are both replacing carbs in a low-carb diet).

The main reason why increasing your protein intake is helpful for weight loss is that on a calorie-for-calorie basis, protein is more satiating than both carbs and fat. This means that if your protein intake is high, you can eat less food than normal without feeling any hungrier.

Protein also has a higher "thermic effect of food" than the other macronutrients, which simply means that it takes more energy (i.e. calories) for your body to digest protein than to digest carbs or fat.

Finally, when weight is lost on a high-protein diet, the lost weight will come more from burning stored bodyfat than from losing muscle tissue, because a high protein intake protects lean muscle during a calorie deficit. This will benefit you even if you don't want to actually *build* muscle; you'll simply lose more fat, rather than losing both fat and healthy, lean muscle tissue.

The good news is that the paleo diet tends to be naturally high in protein by default, especially with a low-carb paleo diet, so your protein intake may already be pretty good. However, because many paleo foods are high in healthy fats, for weight loss it may be helpful to focus a bit more on keeping your protein intake high and keeping your fat intake more moderate.

This may mean pulling back a bit on some foods that are low in protein but high in fat (avocados, healthy oils, nut butters, ghee, tallow, bacon fat, etc) and focusing more on foods that contain relatively higher amounts of protein (most notably meat and eggs). You may even want to start eating leaner cuts of meat than usual if you normally eat very fatty meats (for example, cutting down on the bacon and eat more chicken breasts).

As a rough rule of thumb, your protein intake for maximum weight loss should be about 1 gram of protein for every pound of your "ideal" bodyweight. For example, if your target bodyweight is 150 lbs, you should be eating about 150 grams of protein per day. This amount of protein is pretty high for most people, and requires you to make protein-rich foods like meat the main part of every meal you eat, but it's very effective.

Note that you shouldn't cut back on your fat intake too harshly when increasing your protein intake; the healthy fats found in paleo foods are absolutely vital for good health. The takeaway here is simply that if you're eating a very high-fat diet, you may want to dial it back to a more moderate fat intake while adding in more healthy, whole-food protein sources.

Don't forget exercise

For the vast majority of people, changing their diet is a much more effective way to lose weight than changing their exercise habits. In fact, most people can lose a lot of weight with diet alone and zero exercise.

That being said, engaging in healthy, low-intensity physical activity on a regular basis provides a great foundation for fat loss by helping to burn some extra calories and keep your body healthy overall. It's something you should be doing for your general healthy and wellbeing anyway, so if you haven't yet gotten around to making healthy exercise a regular habit, now is a good time to start! Not only will it help with your overall health, it will also help a bit with your weight loss. For details on paleo exercise principles, see the chapters on Low Intensity Exercise and Higher Intensity Exercise.

Cut carbs more strictly

Some people find that for whatever reason, the guidelines for carb intake listed above aren't quite strict enough for them. You may need to lower your carb intake because you're smaller than the average person. You may be one of those people who anecdotally seems more prone to gain weight from eating carbs. You may even be inaccurately estimating your carb intake, and consuming more than you think!

Whatever the reason, it's worth a try to knock your carb intake down a bit. Start with eliminating roughly 25-50 grams of carbs per day (depending on how many you're eating now), or simply cut out some carb-based foods like fruit, and see if it makes a difference.

Clear out your pantry

It's pretty common for many people who have *mostly* switched to the paleo diet to still have some unhealthy food lying around in their house. It may be for occasional snacking, it may be "comfort food" to eat after a particularly stressful day, or you may just not have gotten around to clearing out your cupboards in a while. For whatever reason, many people who eat paleo still have chips, candy, soda, bread, or other non-paleo items stashed in their kitchen, despite the fact that their diet is mostly paleo.

Having some non-paleo food around isn't always an issue, but in some cases it can be a bit of a problem, particularly if you have a history of struggling to lose weight. Having junk food in the house will tempt you to stray from your healthy eating habits, simply because it's there, ready and waiting and convenient. And even though occasional indulges are fine, and not something to beat yourself up about, indulging on a regular basis can really throw off your healthy eating habits, and potentially stall weight loss.

The bad news is that if you live with people who aren't paleo, you aren't really going to be able to implement this strategy (unless you get them to go paleo with you!). The good news is that if you're able to clear out your pantry, the simple habit of not keeping any unhealthy food in your house makes it surprisingly easy to consistently eat healthy. As long as you've got at least a few convenient, easy to prepare paleo meals and snacks on hand, you'll find that you're much less tempted to eat junk food, since getting that junk food becomes much more inconvenient.

So if it's possible with your living situation, go clear your pantry out right now: don't worry about things like wasting a few dollars worth of food you haven't finished (consider it a "health tax"), not having snacks for your non-paleo friends (they'll understand that you're trying to be healthy), or other concerns. We think you'll find that clearing out the last of the junk food from your house is a surprisingly liberating experience!

"Cheat" less often

The flip side of the above point is that some people may find that, although they're being very consistent in keeping their diet paleo at home, they may find themselves in other situations in which they're "cheating" a bit more often than they should be.

It's certainly fine to indulge occasionally, or to go "off your diet" in certain situations: if you're celebrating a birthday party with a friend, go ahead and have some birthday cake! Just be sure that these occasional compromises don't creep into your diet too often, otherwise you may be compromising your diet more than you realize.

People often allow themselves to eat extra junk food in situations where it isn't really a necessary compromise; you may get a burger and fries when you're out at a restaurant with your friends (because it's cheaper than getting the steak with veggies), buy yourself a candy bar at the office (because it's more convenient than making your own paleo power bars at home), etc. Each of these little compromises is fine in and of itself, but over time they can add up to a significant amount of extra calories, carbs, refined sugars, and other substances that interfere with weight loss.

Again, we definitely don't recommend that you become neurotic about your eating habits! But if you're the type of dieter that regularly allows yourself to "cheat", you may want to re-evaluate your regular eating habits and try to come up with some easy, enjoyable, and more paleo-friendly replacements for your current list of "cheat" foods.

Check your body composition,

not your scale weight

Most of us have been conditioned to think about our body composition primarily in terms of how much we weigh, and not so much in terms of more relevant factors like our bodyfat percentage, blood work, etc. Even the language we use to talk about our bodies is misleading: the term we all use to refer to losing fat is "losing weight", and our doctors talk to us about keeping ourselves within a "healthy weight range".

On closer examination, this focus on weight is silly. After all, we all know that there's a huge difference between a guy who weighs two hundred pounds because he's skinny but very tall, a guy who weighs two hundred pounds because he has huge muscles, and a guy who weighs two hundred pounds because he's morbidly obese. And to use an even more obvious example, if "losing weight" was really all that we were interested in, you could easily lose twenty or thirty pounds immediately by simply cutting off one of your arms!

The takeaway here is that if you think you aren't making progress because you aren't losing *weight* as quickly as you'd like, you may want to take a step back and look at the whole picture.

For example, if the scale isn't budging, but you feel better and seem to be noticing differences in your appearance, you may simply be losing some fat and *gaining* some muscle. This is particularly easy to miss if you still have a decent amount of bodyfat, since your bodyfat will hide the new muscle you're gaining. This can discourage people in the beginning phase of a diet and exercise program, because they think they haven't made any progress, when they're actually making perfectly good progress without realizing it.

Another example occurs when people think their weight loss has "slowed down". This is often a result of the fact that when a person first starts going on a diet and losing weight (particularly a low carb diet), much of the weight they're losing is water weight, not bodyfat. The initial water weight gets lost quickly, making it seem like weight loss is slowing down once the excess water is gone. This can discourage people into thinking they're doing something wrong, when in actual fact they're simply settling into a healthy, steady, normal rate of fat loss.

So before you jump to conclusions because your scale is telling you that you aren't losing weight, be sure to balance that abstract, context-free, isolated number on the scale against other factors, like the way you look in the mirror, the way your muscles feel, how recently you began your weight loss journey, etc. "Weight" isn't everything!

Manage your stress

Many people don't realize it, but stress isn't just a purely emotional phenomenon. Experiencing stress causes your body to produce increased levels of the hormone cortisol, the "fight-or-flight" hormone that your body only naturally produces in emergency situations.

In small, occasional doses cortisol is perfectly fine, such as during periods of intense exercise. But when you're stressed on a regular basis (as a result of financial, personal, emotional, or other issues), the resulting chronic increase in cortisol can have serious negative health consequences. This includes breaking down and weakening healthy lean muscle tissue, worsening insulin sensitivity, and (most relevant to this discussion) promoting the storage of bodyfat. It can also interfere with your sleep quality, which is another contributing factor to obesity.

The good news is that reducing stress is something that most of us would really like to do anyway! So if you feel like you're regularly stressed out, but haven't had the time or motivation to actively do anything about it, having the added goal of losing weight gives you the perfect reason to get started.

The exact methods that you use to deal with stress are up to you; people benefit from a range of strategies, including meditation, massage, calming exercise like tai chi or yoga, nature walks, etc. You're encouraged to experiment with any and all stress-reducing activities that appeal to you; whatever you choose to do, if it reduces your stress, it will help you not only lose weight, but also just lead a happier, more stress-free life!

Get more (and better) sleep

At first glance, it doesn't seem like sleeping habits and weight loss should have anything to do with each other. After all, every behavior that contributes to weight loss (like diet and exercise) takes place while you're awake. However, the connection between sleep habits and weight gain/loss has been studied fairly extensively, and the conclusions are clear: bad sleeping habits tend to lead to weight gain.

A number of large-scale observational studies have linked lack of sleep to increased bodyfat, and science has discovered that the reason for this is hormonal. Sleep is a critical time for your body's production of all kinds of hormones, and it affects two hormones that play a key role in weight management: ghrelin and leptin. Ghrelin and leptin regulate your appetite; ghrelin is the "go" hormone that tells you when to eat, and leptin is the "stop" hormone that tells you when to stop eating.

Studies have shown that one of the effects of sleep-deprivation is to increase your body's production of ghrelin and decrease its production of leptin. This means that, although missing out on sleep doesn't directly affect your bodyfat, it does trigger a hormonal response that makes you more hungry and prone to overeat, which in turns causes the weight gain.

This doesn't mean that the more you sleep, the more weight you'll lose; getting more (and better) sleep only benefits you up to the point where your sleep is "optimized". For example, if you currently sleep eight hours a night, sleeping an extra half hour a night isn't going to make you drop that last ten pounds. However, if you're only sleeping six hours a night, and start increasing it to seven or eight, you'll almost certainly start to see some extra weight coming off from this one factor alone.

So if you've been skimping on sleep lately for whatever reason, you may want to consider taking a second look at your sleeping habits – not only will good sleep improve your overall health, but it will help your weight loss efforts as well. See the chapter on Sleep for guidelines.

Cut down on "healthy" processed foods

There are a fairly large number of processed or semi-processed foods on the market which are actually pretty paleo-friendly. Common examples you can find in most grocery and health food stores include beef jerky, many energy bars, bottled drinks (coconut water, fruit juice, kombucha), gluten-free bread or noodles, sweet potato chips, pre-made condiments (salsa, ketchup, guacamole), prepared meats like sausages, and many others.

Most paleo eaters have no trouble with these foods as long as they're somewhat careful about reading labels. However, if you find yourself eating these types of pre-packaged, semi-processed foods as the majority of your diet, you may be introducing some unhealthy food additives into your diet without realizing it.

Many of these products contain at least some added sugar, even if the food itself isn't sweet (for example, condiments like ketchup and salsa, or prepared meats like sausage). The same goes for foods that are artificially sweetened (most commonly diet sodas), which don't technically contain any calories or carbs, but which may have other ingredients that negatively affect your appetite, digestive bactieria, etc.

If your diet consists largely of "products" (even low-carb products), you may want to consider backing off a bit on the pre-packaged stuff and instead shifting to a diet based more around real, whole foods that you prepare yourself at home. "Natural" foods aren't magic, but eating a diet based around unprocessed whole foods simply helps ensure that you're taking in a diet rich in micronutrients, and avoiding empty calories and unnecessary food additives that may be sneakily creeping into your diet and interfering with weight loss.

Try food journaling

Food journaling is a more mainstream tactic employed by people looking to lose weight and get in shape, and simply involves keeping a record of all the food you eat in a given day, along with the corresponding calories and macronutrients that go with it. This is a bit of a last resort for most paleo eaters, because one of the benefits of adopting a paleo diet is that most people can get down to a lean, healthy weight relatively easily without ever needing to track their food intake. However, there's nothing wrong with food journaling; the only reason not to do it is because it's a pain, and usually unnecessary, not because there are no benefits to doing it.

This means that for people who have firmly adopted a paleo lifestyle, tried losing weight, and not gotten the results they wanted, it can sometimes be helpful to at least temporarily keep a food journal in order to track how many calories and macronutrients they're consuming on a daily basis. This can potentially help reveal little problems or oversights that have cropped up in your diet which may be compromising fat loss without you realizing it.

For example, some people start consuming lots of healthy food on the paleo diet, but because the foods they choose are fairly calorie-dense, they're still eating a calorie surplus at the end of the day. You can lose weight without counting calories, but that doesn't mean calories don't count! It's particularly easy to overeat with healthy fatty foods like coconut products, nuts, avocados, etc, since fat is very calorie-dense. So making sure that you aren't taking in more calories than you thought is a good double-check.

Another common example is that a person eats what they think is a low-carb diet, but since they're only roughly estimating how much carbohydrate they're eating, they may be off by a significant amount. Fifty grams of carbs is enough to change the "weight loss zone" you're in, and this relatively small amount of carbohydrate can sneak up on you sometimes, depending on your eating habits (a tablespoon of honey and a piece of fruit, for example, can easily contribute fifty grams of carbs to your diet). The same goes for underestimating how much protein you're consuming (remember that high protein intake promotes fat loss).

Finally, without taking an objective look at your overall diet, you may be letting a bit more junk food into your diet than you realize. A cookie here, a bagel there, a few pieces of candy from the candy bowl at work … your brain isn't very good at remembering these small indulgences, but sometimes they can really add up over the course of weeks and months.

If you decide that you'd like to give this a try, you can either use one of the many food-tracking websites or apps out there (many of them free to use), or simply jot it down yourself in a text file on your computer or a simple notebook. It will be a little bit of a pain, because you'll have to be fairly thorough about recording the exact amounts of everything you eat and drink, and you'll also have to look up the calorie and macronutrient content for each type of food. You'll also have to be brutally honest about confronting your own eating habits: no more hiding from the little snacks and bits of junk food that you add into your diet throughout the week!

The upside is that you'll only need to keep this journal for a few weeks in order to get a pretty good representative sample of what your normal diet looks like. The paleo diet is designed to be fairly simple, intuitive, and easy to follow; one of the big benefits of paleo is that in the long term, you *don't* have to count calories and track every bite you eat. This is why we're only recommending you try food journaling for a few weeks. At the end of this few weeks, you should have a good idea of what your over all calorie and macronutrient intake is, as well as getting a more objective sense of how well you're sticking to the paleo diet, and from there, it's an easy matter to determine what changes you need to make (if any).

Keep doing what you're doing!

The paleo diet is an extremely effective fat loss method, but it's not necessarily a fat loss *shortcut*. Some people start to see results almost instantly from cutting out carbs, grains, sugars, and vegetable oils, while others may need a few weeks to adjust before the weight starts coming off.

Many people don't realize that weight loss is typically a relatively slow process, and the rate at which people lose weigh on a diet is often pretty irregular. For example, most people who are substantially overweight lose a pretty significant amount of weight when they first start a paleo diet, but after this initial burst their weight loss slows down pretty significantly.

Some of this is a result of losing "water weight" in the first stage of your new diet, and some of it is just a natural part of your body adjusting to the fact that it's losing its fat stores. Your body is evolutionarily programmed to conserve energy and hold onto stored bodyfat as an emergency supply of calories in times of famine, so it will try to defend these fat stores if it can.

It's also true that the more weight you lose, the slower you'll lose additional weight in the future. It's actually very easy to lose 30 lbs when you weigh 300 lbs to start with, but losing even 10 lbs is much more difficult when you're around your "ideal bodyweight". If you've lost a fair amount of weight, but would like to continue losing weight, you'll just have to be content with a slower rate of progress than you had in the beginning.

It can be discouraging to feel like you're doing everything right and still not losing as much weight as you want. But sometimes this type of plateau isn't caused by you making any mistakes, it's just a normal part of the journey. You should definitely use the above list of troubleshooting strategies to double-check your habits and make sure you aren't accidentally doing anything to undermine your weight loss plan! But if you've carefully double-checked all your weight loss habits and determined that you're doing everything right, you may just need to accept the fact that reaching your desired bodyweight is simply going to take more time, patience, and consistency over the long term. So if you're doing everything you're supposed to be doing, all that's left is to hang in there and make it happen!

Qualitative Guidelines for Cutting Carbs (Without Counting)

To determine what foods you should base your diet around for various levels of carb restriction, here's a rough guideline you can use to qualitatively restrict the amount of carbs in your diet without actually counting carbs:

- Least amount of carb restriction that will produce consistent fat loss: foods to eat include meat, fish, eggs, organ meats, vegetables, healthy oils, nuts, seeds, some fruit, very small amounts of sweet potatoes and yams, and possibly very small amounts of paleo sweeteners (honey or maple syrup).

- Slightly more carb restriction: foods include meat, fish, eggs, organs, vegetables, healthy oils, nuts, seeds, and some fruit.

- Even more carb restriction: foods include meat, fish, eggs, organs, vegetables, healthy oils, nuts, and seeds.

- Highest level of carb restriction: foods include meat, fish, eggs, organs, vegetables, and healthy oils.

A few notes to keep in mind with the above guidelines:

- Paleo-friendly artificial sweeteners (stevia and xylitol) can also be included in the above plans, since they contain virtually no calories or carbs.

- Grass-fed butter can be included as a healthy fat, even though it's technically dairy, if you're comfortable including it as part of your paleo diet.

- Non-sweet fruits (like tomatoes and avocados) can safely be counted as "vegetables" for the purposes of the above list, since they're extremely low in carbs.

- If you're eating sweet potatoes, paleo sweeteners like honey or maple syrup, or even fruit, these carb sources should ideally be consumed after exercise, so that the glucose in these foods goes towards replacing lost muscle glycogen (rather than stored as fat).

- Herbs and spices have no calories or macronutrients, so they can obviously be used as much as you want.

Equipment Guidelines

To make the majority of the recipes in this book, the basic equipment you will need is:

- A food processor.

- A few saucepans and frying pans.

- An oven-safe baking dish or pan (and parchment paper to line it, for a few recipes).

- Measuring cups and spoons.

If you don't have them, these items can all be purchased very cheaply: in fact, it's recommended that when you're first starting out, you buy the cheapest versions of these items you can find (the cheap versions work just fine, and you can decide later if you want to save up your pennies for a more expensive model).

There are also a few more specialized pieces of equipment, which are technically optional, but are helpful (or sometimes even necessary) for certain recipes. These include:

- Ramekins (to bake and serve individual-serving quiches or custards, if desired).

- A microplane (a handheld grater, commonly used to make lime/lemon/orange zest, and which can also be used to grate fresh ginger or cinnamon sticks).

- A muffin tin or tins, as well as muffin liners.

- A blender (primarily for one smoothie recipe, although also useful for preparing sauces, dressings, marinades, etc).

- A large stock pot.

- A cooling rack / cake rack.

- A slow cooker / crock pot.

These items, while somewhat more specialized, can also be obtained very inexpensively if you shop around a bit, and will usually last for years with proper care.

Finally, for non-U.S. readers, note that since this book was originally published for the American market, all measurements are based on the U.S. system (weight in pounds, temperature in degrees Fahrenheit, etc). We apologize for the slight inconvenience this causes; luckily, online calculators makes it quick and easy it to convert these measurements to whatever system you use in your home country.

Ingredient Discussion

The vast majority of the ingredients used in the recipes in this book are self-explanatory, and almost all are commonplace in paleo cooking. However, there are some ingredients that require a little more explanation; some of them aren't widely agreed on as being strictly paleo, and some of them simply require clarification regarding where they should be sourced, how they should be used, etc.

If you have any questions about the ingredients used in any of the recipes in this book, there's a good chance your questions will be answered below. If there are any ingredients not covered in this section that you're unsure about, they can usually be easily looked up with a quick internet search.

Butter

Butter is technically not paleo. Our hunter-gatherer ancestors didn't consume dairy in any form, which is why many paleo plans omit butter altogether.

However, this book includes butter in a number of recipes, with the expectation that you can substitute it for something else if you're a strict purist when it comes to dairy (more on that in a moment).

The reason butter is included here as a paleo ingredient is that, although butter isn't technically paleo, it's composition happens to be very similar to the ancestral foods we evolved to eat. The fat found in grass-fed butter is very similar to the actual fat tissue of ruminant animals (cows, goats, etc), and contains a number of health-promoting nutrients. This includes CLA (a healthy fat that has been linked to benefits to cardiovascular health, reducing the risk of certain cancers, and fat loss), butyrate (a short-chain fatty acid shown to be anti-inflammatory), vitamins A, D, E, and K2, and a perfect 1:1 ratio of Omega 6 to Omega 3 fatty acids. For these reasons, butter is included here as a healthy, mostly-paleo ingredient.

If you're a strict paleo purist (or extremely sensitive to lactose, casein, etc), and don't want to consume any dairy whatsoever, butter can usually be replaced with either coconut butter or coconut oil (depending on the recipe). For a compromise approach, you can also experiment with using ghee, a type of "clarified butter" that is 100% pure butterfat, rendered down so that all lactose and dairy proteins have been completely removed.

When using any of these foods as a substitute for "normal" butter, be sure to experiment with the recipe carefully to ensure that the change in ingredients doesn't negatively impact the taste or texture of the dish.

And finally, be sure to use *grass-fed* butter, not conventional, factory-farmed butter from grain-fed cows. If you aren't sure where to get butter that's grass-fed, a common (and highly recommended) brand that you can find in most grocery stores is Kerrygold. Kerrygold is an Irish company that unfortunately doesn't list on the label that it's butter is from grass-fed cows. However, not only is this brand grass-fed, it's also widely lauded for its excellent taste and texture.

Remember, the above-mentioned health benefits of butter only apply if it's grass-fed! So if you can't find butter from grass-fed cows, you might want to skip it altogether and use a more paleo-friendly substitute.

Salt

Generally speaking, you can use any type of salt in you cooking, however sea salt is probably the ideal choice. Regular table salt is simply composed of pure sodium chloride (sometimes with added iodine), which is one of the four natural electrolytes. However, sea salt contains all four types of electrolytes (sodium, potassium, magnesium, and calcium), making it a bit healthier than regular table salt.

You can use any type of salt you prefer for the recipes in this book, but whenever "salt" is listed as an ingredient, it's assumed that you'll be using natural sea salt.

Coconut Milk

Whenever a recipe in this book calls for "coconut milk", this refers to the type of minimally processed full-fat coconut milk sold in cans for cooking, as opposed to the processed, flavored coconut milks often sold in cartons for use as beverages. Th ingredients listed on the can should usually read something like "Coconut, Water, Guar Gum" (and nothing else).

This is an important distinction: if you use "light" coconut milk, or the thin, processed coconut milk sold in cartons, it will probably negatively affect the recipe. All the recipes in this book that list "coconut milk" as an ingredient call for full-fat canned coconut milk .

Cocoa Powder (and Chocolate)

When the term "cocoa powder" is used in a recipe, this specifically refers to pure, 100% cacao, unsweetened cocoa powder. Some cocoa powders have added sugar, flavorings, etc; be sure to avoid these, since they're less healthy than pure chocolate powder, and also completely unnecessary from a culinary standpoint (every recipe that uses cocoa powder also includes natural sweeteners and flavorings).

Also, be sure to avoid any chocolate that has been "Dutch processed" or "alkalized"; these terms (which should be listed on the packaging if they were used) refer to processes that lighten the color of chocolate and remove some of the bitter flavor. Unfortunately, they also remove most of the beneficial antioxidant content of the chocolate. To avoid this, be sure to choose a brand of cocoa powder that is either raw or roasted.

Nightshades

A number of recipes in this book use plants in the "nightshade" family, like tomatoes and bell peppers, as ingredients. For some people who are particularly strict about the paleo diet, nightshades are frowned on because they technically contain small amounts of harmful compounds, like lectins and alkaloids. Additionally, some people seem to have food sensitivities to these plants.

Nightshades are included in these recipes simply because most people who follow the paleo lifestyle are comfortable with them. The levels of problematic compounds found in common foods like tomatoes are very low, and there is currently no available research linking these common foods to bad health. So for most people, enjoying a dish that includes some diced tomatoes or bell peppers isn't a big deal.

However, if you're following a more strict version of the paleo diet, or if you find that you are particularly sensitive to nightshades, feel free to modify any recipe in this book that uses tomatoes, bell peppers, hot sauce, or similar ingredients by either removing or substituting the problematic ingredient, or avoiding the recipe altogether. And remember that personal experimentation will be the best way to determine what feels best for you.

A Note on Animal Products

Meat and animal products are used throughout this book. Please note that, although animal products from any source will work, for the sake of your health you should ideally be using animal products from pasture-raised animals. This means grass-fed cows, pasture-raised chickens (different from "cage-free"), pigs raised in open pens with room to move, and wild-caught seafood.

Again, from a culinary standpoint, any type of animal products can be used and the recipes will still turn out delicious! But there's a reason why every paleo health expert under the sun recommends pasture-raised animal products: they have a better fatty acid profile, lower levels of environmental toxins, and are consistently higher in micronutrients than their factory-farmed counterparts. Pasture-based or wild-caught animal products are better for animal welfare, better for the environment, and better for your health!

A Note on Artificial Sweeteners

Although there are a wide range of artificial sweeteners on the market, two in particular are of interest to health-conscious practitioners of the paleo diet: stevia and xylitol. Each of these is discussed in more detail below.

It should be noted that any of the recipes in this book that call for artificial sweeteners are based on approximate amounts. If you're new to using these sweeteners, you should experiment with both the type of sweetener you're using, the particular form it comes in (for example, liquid vs. powder), the brands you choose, and finally the amount of sweetener used in the actual recipe itself.

The amounts listed in any recipe in this book are simply recommended starting points, not set in stone. You should most certainly do your own experimentation to find out what you like best!

Stevia

Stevia is a popular non-caloric sweetener among many health-conscious people, and often used as an alternative to conventional artificial sweeteners like sucralose (mostly commonly known under the brand name Splenda) and aspartame (the sweetener used in most diet sodas). Stevia is derived from a South American herb, and can be purchased in either powder or liquid form.

Studies on stevia have linked it to a number of health benefits, including increasing insulin sensitivity and decreasing post-meal blood sugar levels. In fact, the Japanese have been using stevia to treat type 2 diabetics for decades for exactly this reason. This also makes stevia particularly appealing for low-carb dieters, who are usually trying to reduce blood sugar and increase insulin sensitivity as much as possible.

Stevia is very sweet, and perfectly healthy for anyone to use. The one drawback is that many people complain that it has a very distinct, unpleasant underlying flavor. Some people claim that this is simply an acquired taste, that you'll get used to after a while, while some say they simply can't get used to it.

If you're interested in experimenting with Stevia, try multiple brands, as well as both the powdered and liquid forms.

Xylitol

Xylitol is the most popular member of the family of artificial sweeteners derived from sugar alcohols, and boasts a number of benefits over other artificial sweeteners that make it popular with the health crowd.

First, it has very little effect on blood glucose levels, and no effect on insulin levels, making it another excellent choice for diabetics, low-carb dieters, and anyone else concerned with managing their blood sugar and insulin.

Second, unlike almost any other sweetener, xylitol actually *protects* your teeth, with a number of studies showing that it has a protective effect against dental plaque and cavities. It's even included as an active ingredient in many natural/organic toothpastes.

The only potential downside to using xylitol is that if you eat too much, too soon, it might give you mild diarrhea. This is because your body needs to adapt its digestive enzymes to consuming it; if you're going to use it regularly, consume it sparingly for the first few weeks to give your body time to adjust.

Lamb and Bacon Meatballs

Ingredients

Meatballs

1 lb ground lamb

6 slices bacon

½ small white onion, finely chopped

1 large egg

2 tsp chopped fresh sage

1 tsp paprika

Salt and pepper to taste

Sauce

3 cups diced fresh tomatoes

1 tsp basil, finely chopped

Salt and pepper to taste

Directions

Meatballs

1. Preheat oven to 350 F.

2. Heat a frying pan over medium heat, add bacon, and cook until done. Remove from pan, allow to cool, and then finely dice, reserving bacon grease in pan.

3. Saute onion in bacon fat until translucent. Remove from pan and allow to cool.

4. In a large bowl, combine all meatball ingredients and mix well. Roll the mixture into balls of desired size (1½-2 inches in diameter works well).

5. Transfer balls to a baking dish and bake for 30-40 minutes, or until well cooked.

Sauce

1. Combine all sauce ingredients in a saucepan over medium heat and mix well. Bring to a simmer, and simmer for 2-3 minutes.

2. Meatballs can be added to the saucepan and simmered for another 5-10 minutes before serving, or sauce simply can be drizzled over meatballs and served warm.

Notes

- If convenient, you can also use canned diced tomatoes to make the sauce (rather than fresh ones). The taste won't be as fresh, but since the canned tomatoes are already cooked (as part of the canning process, they will be easier to make sauce out of. You can even opt to avoid cooking the canned version of the sauce in the first place: simply combine all ingredients in a food processor and blend to desired consistency (just remember to warm it up by your preferred method before serving).

Ginger Beef and Broccoli

Ingredients

1 lb beef stew meat, cubed

2 cups broccoli florets

2 cups carrots, thinly sliced

1 green onion, thinly sliced

½-¾ cup chicken broth

2 cloves garlic, crushed

2 Tbsp lemon juice

2 tsp grated fresh ginger root

2 tsp freshly ground black pepper

½ tsp. red pepper flakes

Cooking oil

1. Heat a frying pan over medium-high heat and coat with oil. Add beef to pan and cook, turning frequently, until browned on all sides. Remove from pan and drain excess beef juices.

2. Return pan to heat, reduce heat to medium, and coat with more cooking oil if necessary.

3. In a bowl, combine lemon juice, ginger, black pepper, and red pepper flakes with ½ cup of chicken broth.

4. Add broccoli and carrots to pan, and pour broth mixture over veggies to coat. Cook until broccoli is tender.

5. Return beef to the pan, and add green onions. If necessary, add another ¼ cup chicken broth to ensure that beef is covered in liquid. Allow to simmer gently for a few minutes, until beef is warmed (but not cooked any further). Serve warm.

The first thing that most paleo dieters miss when cutting carbs out of their diet are starchy foods like potatoes. Luckily, there's a great alternative: turnips! Boiled turnips and boiled potatoes have a similar mild flavor and soft texture, making it a great substitution option. And a cup of boiled, cubed turnips only has about 8 grams of carbs, as opposed to the 40 or so grams you'd get from using potatoes.

So if you're craving potatoes, this creamy, crunchy "potato salad" recipe is a great low carb twist on a classic potato recipe that your family will love.

Ingredients

4-5 cups peeled and diced turnips
2-3 hard-boiled eggs, peeled and roughly chopped
1 cup chopped celery

4-6 slices cooked bacon, chopped
1/3 cup Paleo Mayonnaise (see recipe in this book)
2 tsp paprika
1 Tbsp fresh chives, chopped
1 Tbsp fresh parsley
2 tsp fresh dill, chopped
Salt and pepper to taste

Directions

1. Bring a large saucepan of salted water to a boil. Add diced turnips and reduce to medium-high heat. Boil turnips until tender (about 5 minutes).

2. Remove turnips from heat, drain, and set aside to cool.

3. In a large bowl, combine turnips and celery and mix well.

4. Add mayo, bacon, and seasonings and mix again until thoroughly combined.

5. Lastly, sprinkle chopped hard-boiled egg over mixture; you can leave this crumbled egg on top of the dish as a garnish, or gently mix it in with the rest of the salad. Season with additional salt and pepper to taste if desired. Serve at room temperature or chilled.

Broiled Salmon with Rosemary Mustard Sauce

Ingredients

1 salmon fillet (about 6 ounces)

2 fresh lemon slices

Juice of 1 Lemon (after removing above slices)

1 Tbsp Dijon mustard

1 tsp finely chopped fresh rosemary

Salt and pepper to taste

Directions

1. Preheat oven broiler.

2. In a bowl, blend lemon juice, mustard, and rosemary and mix well.

3. Place salmon filet in a broiler-safe pan, sprinkle with salt and pepper to taste, top with lemon slices, and place in oven. Broil until salmon is opaque throughout and flakes easily with a fork, about 8-10 minutes.

4. Transfer salmon to a plate, or on top of preferred vegetables (see Notes section), and drizzle with rosemary mustard sauce. Serve warm.

Notes

- This dish pairs well with veggies; try placing it on a bed of greens, or over roast asparagus.

Avocado Herb Omelet

Ingredients

4 eggs

½-1 cup fresh spinach

½-1 small avocado, sliced

1-2 tsp chopped fresh basil

Salt and pepper to taste

Cooking oil

Directions

1. Heat a frying pan over medium heat and coat with cooking oil. Gently saute spinach until slightly wilted, then remove from pan and set aside.

2. In a bowl, whisk the eggs until smooth, then season with salt and pepper to taste, and mix well.

3. Add more cooking oil to pan if necessary. Pour eggs into pan and spread evenly. Immediately begin stirring continuously, allowing uncooked egg to run underneath and cook evenly.

4. When the bottom of the omelet is firm, but the top layer is still slightly moist, remove pan from heat. Add the sauteed spinach and sliced avocado, sprinkle with fresh basil, and season with additional salt and pepper if desired. Fold omelet in half, and slide off onto a plate. Serve warm.

Notes

- If you'd like to experiment with the texture of the omelet a bit, you can try skipping the first step (sauteing the spinach), and simply fold fresh spinach leaves inside the omelet. You'll just need to use a bit less spinach, since raw spinach is mucher larger in volume than cooked spinach.

- You can also incorporate the basil into the egg mixture before cooking, rather than sprinkling it over the contents of the finished omelet.

Spicy Bison Burgers

Ingredients

1 lb ground bison
1-2 jalapeño peppers, chopped

3 cloves garlic, crushed
1 tsp paprika
1 tsp onion powder
Salt and pepper to taste

Directions

1. In a bowl, combine all and mix well. Form into patties (four ¼-lb patties work well, or two ½-lb patties).

2. Ideally, grill over an open flame for 4-5 minutes until cooked to your desired level of doneness, or pan fry if grilling is inconvenient. Serve warm, topped with veggies, guacamole, or hot sauce.

Notes

- To make the burger extra spicy, without adding extra jalapeno peppers (which would obviously make the flavor of the burger more jalapeno-y), leave the seeds in the peppers. Likewise, to make the burger a bit less spicy, remove the seeds from the jalapenos before adding them to the mix.

Spiced Shrimp Skewers

Shrimp have all the same health benefits as other types of seafood (particularly the rich Omega-3 fats that are so good for us), and are extremely flavorful when cooked properly. This easy dish makes a great appetizer before dinner, and is also great for parties.

Ingredients

20 medium shrimp, peeled

20 cherry tomatoes

1 bell pepper (yellow or red, ideally), seeded and cut into rough chunks

3 garlic cloves, crushed

1 tsp paprika

1 tsp cayenne

Cooking oil (olive oil works well)

(optional) juice from 1 lime

Directions

1. Heat cooking oil in a large frying pan over medium flame. Add garlic, paprika, and cayenne, and sauté for one minute while stirring.

2. Reduce heat to low, and add more cooking oil if necessary. Add shrimp, cover, and cook for ten minutes. Shrimp are done when pink.

3. Place shrimp in a small colander and drain excess liquid. Spear shrimp, bell pepper chunks, and cherry tomatoes, alternating each until skewer is full. If desired, drizzle each skewer with fresh lime juice before serving.

Low-Carb Paleo Pasta with Meat Sauce

Ingredients

2 lbs Italian sausage (spicy or mild)
1 spaghetti squash
1 cup (or more to taste) store-bought pasta sauce (plain marinara is ideal)
1 yellow onion, diced
2 garlic cloves, diced

Cooking oil

Directions

Pasta

1. Preheat the oven to 375 F.

2. With a large, sharp knife, cut the squash in half lengthwise so that you have two long halves. Scoop out the seeds and loose pieces in the center.

3. Brush the cooking oil on the inside surface of the squash liberally, then sprinkle on the salt.

4. Place the squash in an oven safe baking dish with the oiled/cut side facing down. Bake for 30-45 minutes, until the edges of the squash are golden brown and the flesh is soft all the way through. Allow to cool.

5. Use a fork to scrape lengthwise down the inside of the spaghetti squash: this will pull out the natural, noodle-like strands of the squash's flesh, which can be treated exactly like normal pasta.

Sauce

1. If sausage is in the form of links, remove casings.

2. Heat a frying pan over medium heat and coat with cooking oil. Crumble sausage into pan, and cook until sausage is lightly browned, but not quite done cooking.

3. Add onion and garlice to pan and saute until onion is translucent and the sausage is fully cooked.

4. Add the pasta sauce and continue cooking for another 3-5 minutes, stirring frequently, until sauce is warm and well mixed. Pour over spaghetti squash noodles and serve warm.

Notes

- When purchasing storebought pasta sauce, be sure to check the label for any ingredients you don't want in your diet!

Ingredients

4 medium turkey cutlets (about 6 oz each)

2 tsp cayenne pepper

1 tsp paprika

1 tsp onion powder

1 tsp garlic powder

1 tsp oregano

Cooking oil (olive oil works well)

Directions

1. Combine all spices and mix well

2. Roll each turkey cutlet in spice mixture until thoroughly coated.

3. Heat cooking oil in a frying pan over medium-high heat. Add turkey and cook for about ten minutes, flipping often, until turkey is done. Serve warm.

Beef Stew

A classic, comforting dinner recipe, perfect for those cold winter nights when you need a hearty home-cooked meal. The potatoes found in many traditional stew recipes have been replaced with butternut sqaush, making this dish paleo-friendly without compromising the classic beef stew's rich flavor and texture.

Ingredients

2 lbs beef stew meat, cubed

2 cups chicken or beef broth

1 small butternut squash, peeled, seeded, and cubed

4 large carrots, peeled and chopped

4 celery stalks, chopped

1 small yellow onion, chopped

2 garlic cloves, crushed

1 tsp oregano

1 sprig fresh rosemary

Salt and pepper to taste

Cooking oil

Directions

1. Heat cooking oil in a large saucepan over medium heat. Add beef and cook until browned evenly on all sides (about 12 minutes).

2. Remove beef from pan, coat pan with additional cooking oil if necessary. Add onion and garlic and saute for about 5 minutes

3. Add carrots, celery, and squash, and continue to sauté for another 5 minutes.

4. Return beef to pan and add broth. Bring to a boil, then cover and reduce heat to low. Add rosemary and oregano, then cover and simmer for 30 minutes. When stew is done, season with salt and pepper to taste and serve warm.

Lamb Mint Burgers

Lamb is an uncommon ingredient, but tasty and very healthy. Most lamb is grass-fed, making it a great choice for the paleo diet, and although it's almost always more expensive than ground beef, it can be a very nice change of pace for any low-carb paleo dieter who eats a lot of meat, particularly since this recipe utilizes the classic pairing of lamb and fresh mint!

Ingredients

1 lb ground lamb

½ cup diced onion (red or white, ideally)

2 cloves garlic, crushed

2 Tbsp chopped fresh mint

2 Tbsp chopped fresh parsley

1 tsp salt

1 tsp black pepper

1 tsp cumin

1 tsp paprika

1 egg

Directions

1. In a bowl, combine all ingredients and mix by hand, until mixture is evenly combined.

2. Form mixture into patties of desired size (four patties of about ¼ lb each or two large ½ lb patties both work well). Place patties in refrigerator and let sit for at least 30 minutes to allow flavors to meld.

3. To cook, grilling is ideal (about 4 minutes per side), but pan frying works as well. Medium-rare (with a little pink in the middle) is generally considered best, or cook to desired level of doneness.

Moroccan Chicken

Ingredients

4 boneless, skinless chicken breasts, cut into rough 1-inch chunks

2 cups chopped broccoli florets

2 cups chopped carrots

¼ cup raisins

¼ cup chicken broth

1 Tbsp cinnamon

2 tsp cumin

1 tsp ginger powder

¼ tsp cayenne

Salt and pepper to taste

Cooking oil (coconut oil works well)

Directions

1. Heat a sauce pan over medium heat and coat with oil. Add chicken and cook, stirring frequently, until chicken is cooked through (about 5-7 minutes).

2. Add the carrots and broccoli (and more cooking oil if necessary), and cook, stirring frequently, until vegetables start to become tender.

3. Add the spices, raisins, and broth, and stir well. Bring liquid to a simmer and cook for another 5 minutes, or until raisins are tender. Remove from heat and serve warm.

Tomato and Bacon Soup

Ingredients

1½ cups diced tomatoes (fresh or canned)

1½ cups vegetable stock

5 slices bacon, diced

1 small white onion, diced

1-2 tsp dried oregano

1 tsp ground paprika

Salt and pepper to taste

Cooking oil

Directions

1. Heat a sauce pan over medium heat and coat with cooking oil. Add onion and bacon and cook, stirring frequently, until bacon is lightly browned.

2. Add oregano and paprika and cook for another 2 minutes.

3. Add tomatoes and vegetable stock. Cover and simmer for 10-15 minutes. Season with salt and pepper to taste and serve warm.

Paleo Shrimp Tacos

A great recipe for lovers of seafood or Mexican cuisine, without the processed tortillas that make most tacos so unhealthy.

Ingredients

1 lb large shrimp, peeled

10–12 large romaine lettuce leaves

½-1 cup store bought salsa (ideally green salsa)

½ red onion, sliced

3 cloves garlic, crushed

1 green bell pepper, sliced

2 cups fresh spinach

½ Tbsp chili powder

1 lime, cut into eighths

Cooking oil

Directions

1. Heat a frying pan over medium heat and coat with cooking oil. Add onion, garlic, and bell peppers and saute until peppers are tender, about 3-4 minutes.

2. Add shrimp and sauté until shrimp are pink, about 3 minutes.

3. Add the chili powder and salsa and stir well. Cook until salsa is gently warmed.

4. Scoop mixture into lettuce leaves, dividing evenly, top with spinach, and serve with lime wedges.

Egg Muffins

Ingredients

12 large eggs, whisked

½-1 lb breakfast sausage
1 small white onion, finely chopped
1 green or red bell pepper, finely chopped
½ tsp black pepper
¼ tsp salt

Cooking oil

Directions

1. If sausage is in the form of links, remove casings. Preheat oven to 350 F.

2. Heat a frying pan over medium heat and coat with cooking oil. Crumble sausage into pan, and cook until sausage is lightly browned, but not quite done cooking.

3. Add onion to pan and saute until onion is translucent and the sausage is fully cooked. Add bell peppers and for another 2-3 minutes.

4. Once onions/peppers are cooked, transfer to a bowl and allow to cool for a few minutes.

5. Add whisked eggs to bowl and stir well, sprinkling in the salt and pepper.

6. Coat a large muffin pan with cooking oil, then fill each cup evenly with egg mixture. Place in oven and bake for 10–15 minutes. Remove once the tops of the muffins are fluffy and golden brown.

Notes

- For oddly shaped implements like muffin tins, a cooking spray is often convenient for coating with cooking oil. Olive oil (i.e. paleo-friendly) cooking sprays can be purchased online and at many grocery stores.

- If you're having trouble removing the muffins from the tin when they're done baking, you can use a butter knife to gently pop them out – if they don't come out easily, try coating the muffin tin with more cooking oil next time!

- Bacon is another great meat to use with these muffins: just substitute the sausage in the above recipe for 6-8 slices of bacon, cooked and diced before you add it to the egg mixture.

- If you like your eggs a little spicy, you can add hot sauce, tabasco, or sriracha to the mix, and/or chop up a jalapeno pepper and cooking it with the other veggies.

Paleo Veggie Quiche

Ingredients

12 large eggs
½ cup almond flour
1 cup onions, chopped
1 cup spinach, rinsed
½ cup diced red bell pepper, diced small
½ cup diced green bell pepper, diced small
1 tsp baking powder
¼ tsp black pepper, freshly ground

Cooking oil (butter works well)

Directions

1. Preheat oven to 350 F.

2. In a large bowl, whisk eggs, then stir in almond flour and baking powder.

3. Heat a fying pan over medium heat and coat with cooking oil. Add onions and spinach and saute until onions are translucent. Remove from heat and allow to cool briefly.

4. Combine all ingredients and mix well. Pour the mixture into a baking dish and sprinkle lightly with pepper. Bake for 45 minutes, or until a knife inserted into the quiche comes out clean.

Notes

- Just like any egg recipe, this quiche goes really well with bacon or sausage (either served alongside, or mixed into the quiche itself).

- This is a great recipe to make in advance, keep in the fridge, and then grab a slice or two on the go when you're having a hectic morning and need a quick breakfast.

Garlic Chili Chicken Skewers

Although the instructions here are for the more convenient pan-fried version of the recipe, these mouth-watering chicken skewers are perfect for grilling the next time you're having a barbecue.

Ingredients

2 medium chicken breasts, cut into rough 1-inch chunks

6 wooden skewers

4 cloves garlic, crushed

5 Tbsp lemon juice

2 Tbsp olive oil

1-3 tsp chopped red chillies (depending on preferred level of spiciness)

Directions

1. Preheat oven to 350 F.

2. In a small bowl, combine olive oil, chilies, garlic and lemon juice and mix well.

3. Thread diced chicken on skewers and place on an oven tray lined with baking paper. Drizzle garlic chili sauce over the chicken, coating well.

4. Bake in for 35-40 minutes, or until chicken has cooked through.

Notes

- If grilling, the chicken should be cooked for about 5-6 minutes per side.

Thai Chicken Omelet

Ingredients

¼ lb cooked chicken breast, shredded

3 eggs, beaten

1/3 cup bean sprouts

¼ cup shredded carrots

2 green onions, sliced

1 clove garlic, crushed

½ tsp paprika

Salt and pepper to taste

Cooking oil (coconut oil works well)

Directions

1. Heat a frying pan over medium heat and coat with cooking oil. Add onion and garlic and saute until onion is translucent and garlic is fragrant. Remove from pan and set aside.

2. In a bowl, whisk the eggs until smooth, then add paprika and season with salt and pepper to taste and mix well.

3. Add more cooking oil to pan if necessary. Pour eggs into pan and spread evenly. Immediately begin stirring continuously, allowing uncooked egg to run underneath and cook evenly.

4. When the bottom of the omelet is firm, but the top layer is still slightly moist, remove pan from heat. Add chicken, cooked onion and garlic mixture, and fresh carrots and bean sprouts. Fold omelet in half, then gently slide off onto a plate. Season with additional salt, pepper, and/or paprika if desired, and serve warm.

Baked Orange Salmon with Pistachio Salsa

Ingredients

Salmon

1½ lbs fresh salmon fillets

Juice of 1 medium orange

2 Tbsp olive oil

3-4 sprigs fresh dill

Salt

Salsa

½-1 cup chopped fresh parsley

½ cup pistachios, shelled

¼ cup chopped shallots

1 Tbsp capers

1 Tbsp olive oil

Directions

1. Preheat oven to 350 F.

2. Rinse the salmon fillet under cold running water and pat dry with a paper towel. Rub salt into the salmon flesh and wrap in aluminum foil along with dill, orange juice, and olive oil. Fold edges of aluminum foil to form a tight package.

3. Salmon can be placed directly on oven rack if desired (just make sure the aluminum package is tight enough not to leak), or placed in an oven safe baking dish. Bake for 20-30 minutes or until salmon is cooked through.

4. To make the salsa, combine parsley, capers, pistachios, shallots, and olive oil and mix well. Transfer to a food processor and pulse gently until desired consistency is reached. Spoon over cooked salmon and serve warm.

Macadamia Herb Chicken

Ingredients

2 cooked chicken breasts, each breast cut into 3 roughly even slices

½ cup macadamia nuts

1/3 cup diced red onion

4 Tbsp chopped fresh chives

1 clove garlic, chopped

1-2 Tbsp olive oil

Salt and pepper to taste

Cooking oil

Directions

1. Heat a frying pan over medium heat and coat with oil. Add garlic and onion and saute until onion is translucent. Remove from heat and allow to cool.

2. Add all ingredients except chicken to a food processor and pulse until desired consistency is reached (a consistency similar to chunky salsa works well).

3. Spoon macadamia herb topping over chicken and serve warm.

Paleo Pesto

A slight variation on the classic basil pesto recipe makes this delectable sauce 100% paleo. Serve over spaghetti squash noodles like a traditional pasta dish, or add it to an array of interesting recipes (like the following one for Pesto Scrambled Eggs!).

Ingredients

2 cups fresh spinach

½ cup olive oil

1/3 cup pine nuts

3 cloves garlic, crushed

Salt and pepper to taste

Directions

1. Combine all ingredients in a food processor or blender and blend to desired consistency (a blender works well for creating a smoother, more liquid consistency, while a food processor is ideal for making a chunky mixture).

Pesto Scrambled Eggs

This flavorful variation on pesto is a great way to add some variety to your morning eggs.

Ingredients

4 eggs
1-2 Tbsp of Paleo Pesto (see previous recipe)

(optional) salt and pepper to taste

Directions

1. In a bowl, whisk the eggs until smooth, then add pesto and salt and pepper to taste (if using) and mix well.

2. Heat a pan over medium-low heat, coat with cooking oil, and add egg mixture. Stir continuously with a spatula while eggs cook, in order to maintain an even consistency.

3. Remove eggs from pan just before desired consistency is reached, since eggs will continue cooking in their own heat for a moment. Serve warm.

Slow Cooker Shredded Pork

This delectable shredded pork recipe is excerpted from our book on paleo slow cooker recipes, *Paleo Slow Cooking*. You'll find that making pulled pork in a slow cooker not only makes the dish extremely easy to make (just throw some ingredients in a slow cooker and you're pretty much done!), but the slow, gentle, lengthy cooking process causes the meat to come out juicy, tender, and extremely flavorful.

If you don't own a slow cooker already, recipes like this are a great reason to get one!

Ingredients

3 lbs pork shoulder

1 can (about 14 oz) tomato sauce

3 Tbsp chili powder

3 Tbs maple syrup

2 tsp coriander

1 tsp cumin

6 cloves garlic, crushed

1 large yellow onion, diced

1/4 cup lime juice (fresh or bottled)

Salt and pepper to taste

Directions

1. In a bowl, combine the tomato sauce, lime juice, maple syrup, chili powder, coriander, and cumin and mix well to form a sauce.

2. Place pork in slow cooker and pour sauce over. Turn the pork shoulder over to evenly coat it with the sauce.

3. Add the garlic and onion, and cook on low for 8-10 hours.

4. Serve by shredding with a fork, and coating with the remaining sauce from the slow cooker if desired.

Notes

- If you're interested in more paleo-friendly slow cooker recipes that are as easy to make as they are delicious, be sure to check out our book *Paleo Slow Cooking!* Click here to check out *Paleo Slow Cooking.*

Paleo Taco Salad

Ingredients

1 lb ground beef
4 cups (or more) chopped romaine lettuce
1 cup sliced or chopped tomatoes
1 cup salsa (homemade or storebought)
½ cup chopped bell peppers (any color)
1 Tbsp chili powder
1 tsp onion powder
1 tsp garlic powder (or 2 cloves of fresh garlic, grated or finely chopped)
1 avocado, sliced
2 limes, halved or quartered

Cooking oil

Directions

1. Heat a frying pan over medium-high heat and coat with oil. Add beef, sprinkle with spices, and cook, stirring frequently until meat is browned. Remove from heat.

2. In a bowl, combine lettuce, tomatoes, and bell peppers and toss until well mix. Top with cooked meat mixture, salsa, and avocado slices, and finally squeeze fresh lime juice on as a light dressing before serving.

Notes

- This recipe also makes a nice paleo "taco": instead of serving over lettuce like a salad, just wrap portions of the meat and toppings in a large romaine lettuce leaf.

- The spice blend used in this recipe is also a great fit for other types of meat: try it with ground turkey, or even more exotic meats like bison.

- If you're a fan of guacamole, add in a big dollop in place of the avocado.

Southwest Smoothie

This unique, low-carb, savory smoothie (excerpted from our book *Paleo Smoothies)* is a great way to easily get in a big dose of your daily vegetables when you're in too much of a hurry to make a salad (or just not in the mood to chew on bowlful of veggies).

Ingredients

2 tomatoes, peeled and chopped

1 cup water

1/2 red pepper, chopped

1/2 cucumber, peeled and chopped

1/2 avocado

1 tsp lemon juice

Dash of black pepper

4-6 ice cubes

Notes

- If your blender isn't high-powered enough to blend this recipe as smoothly as you'd like, you can change the ratio of liquid-to-solid by substituting 1½ cups tomato juice for the 2 tomatoes (just be sure to remove the 1 cup water).

- This nutrient-rich, low-carb smoothie is a sample recipe taken from one of our other paleo recipe books, *Paleo Smoothies*. If you're interested in learning how to make dozens of different healthy, delicious gourmet smoothies, be sure to check it out! Click here to check out *Paleo Smoothies*.

Easy Veggie Frittata

Ingredients

4 eggs
1 large handful fresh spinach, chopped
1 cup diced carrots
¾ cup chopped Portobello mushrooms
½ cup chopped tomato
½ cup finely chopped scallions
1 tsp garlic powder
½ tsp dried thyme
¼ tsp dried rosemary
¼ tsp basil
Salt and pepper to taste

Cooking oil

Directions

1. Preheat oven to 375 F. Grease a 9-inch pie plate or large baking dish with cooking oil.

2. In a bowl, combine all ingredients and mix well. When well combined, pour mixture into pie plate or baking dish.

3. Bake for about 30 minutes, or until a knife inserted into the center of the fritatta comes out clean. Allow to cool briefly, season with additional salt and pepper if desired, and serve warm.

Carrot Zucchini Meatballs

Ingredients

1 pound grass-fed lean ground beef
2 large carrots, diced or shredded
1 small zucchini, diced
½ cup almond flour
¼ cup onion, diced
2 cloves garlic, minced
2 eggs
1 tsp black pepper
1 tsp unrefined sea salt
1 tsp dried oregano
½ tsp fresh cilantro, chopped
½ tsp thyme, chopped

Cooking oil

Directions

1. Preheat oven to 350 F.

2. Heat a frying pan over medium heat and coat with oil. Add garlic and sauté until lightly browned. Add zucchini and carrots and cook until soft, about 3-5 minutes, then remove from heat and allow to cool.

3. In a bowl, combine sauteed veggie mixture and all remaining ingredients and mix well. Shape into meatballs of desired size (1½-2 inches works well). Transfer to a baking sheet

and bake for 25-30 minutes. Serve warm.

Spicy Tuna Salad

1 (6-oz.) cans oil-packed tuna

1 large handful lettuce, spinach, or mixed greens

½ avocado, sliced

1 green onions, chopped

1 jalapeno pepper, chopped

1 Tbsp red chili flakes

1-2 Tbsp lemon juice (ideally fresh)

1 Tbsp olive oil

Directions

1. In a bowl, combine the tuna, green onions, jalapeno pepper, and red chili flakes and mix well.
2. Fill a bowl with greens and top with tuna mixture. Drizzle with olive oil and lemon juice, then top with sliced avocado and serve.

Notes

- To make the salad extra spicy, leave the seeds in the jalapeno peppers. Likewise, to make it a bit less spicy, remove the seeds from the jalapenos before chopping.

- If convenient, you can allow the tuna mixture (made in Step 1) sit in an airtight container in the refrigerator overnight to allow the flavors to meld before eating. Besides subtly improving the flavor of the mixture, this also makes for an easy grab-and-go recipe: just throw the mixture onto a bed of greens, toss with dressing, and you're done.

- If you're interested in tasty, portable paleo meals you can take with you on the go, check out our book *Paleo on the Go* for more!. Click here to check out *Paleo On the Go.*

Lemon and Egg Salad

Ingredients

1-2 cups spinach

2 hard boiled eggs, diced

¼ small red onion, diced

1 celery stalk, finely sliced

1-2 Tbsp pine nuts

1 Tbsp Paleo Mayonnaise (see recipe in this book)

2 tsp lemon juice

Directions

1. In a small bowl, combine paleo mayonnaise and lemon juice and mix well to make the dressing.

2. In a salad bowl, combine all remaining ingredients and mix well. Drizzle with dressing and serve.

Meaty Chef's Salad

This paleo take on a classic salad is a feast of color and texture: juicy, sweet tomatoes, crunchy celery, salty bacon, and fresh, tangy lemon. If you're looking for a big salad you can make a meal out of, this one's hard to beat.

Ingredients

1 head green or red leaf lettuce, chopped

1 avocado, diced

½ lb cooked ham, diced

2-3 slices bacon, cooked and diced

4 large hard-boiled eggs, halved

8 cherry tomatoes, halved

4 green onions, sliced thin

2 stalks celery, diced

1 Tbsp olive oil

Juice of 1 lemon

Directions

1. Divide red leaf lettuce between 2-3 bowls and top with cherry tomatoes, green onions, celery, avocado, eggs, bacon, and ham, dividing evenly.

2. To serve, drizzle with olive oil and fresh lemon juice, and serve at room temperature or chilled. Toss well before eating.

Notes

- If you're planing on making this recipe frequently, you can save quite a bit of time by preparing a sufficient amount of cooked ham and hard-boiled eggs beforehand. Everything else should ideally be prepared just before serving to preserve the flavor, but it's a relatively easy matter to cut up all the veggies in a few minutes while your bacon is cooking!

- To add a little salty bacon flavor to the dish, you can reserve the melted fat from the pan you cook the bacon in and drizzle it over the salad long with the olive oil and lemon juice.

Shrimp Salad

A healthy, delicious, and very simple meal, perfect for lunch on a warm afternoon when you're in the mood for something light and fresh.

Ingredients

1 lb shrimp, boiled, peeled, and (if desired) roughly chopped

2 cups fresh spinach
½ cup Paleo Mayonnaise (see recipe in this book)
2 green onions, sliced
1-2 stalks celery, chopped
2 Tbsp chopped fresh parsley
2 tsp Dijon mustard
1 tsp white wine vinegar

Directions

1. In a bowl, combine all ingredients except spinach and mix well.

2. Place mixture in refrigerator and allow to sit for at least 1 hour to allow flavors to meld.

3. Serve on a bed of fresh spinach, ideally chilled, or at room temperature if desired.

Notes

- This recipe also works well as a wrap (served in large Romaine lettuce leaves), or as an appetizer served on slices of cucumber or zucchini.

Coconut Shrimp

Dishes this exotic and flavorful are rarely this simple to make; luckily, this one's an exception!

Ingredients

1 lb shrimp or prawns (30 to 40 count total), in shell

1 (13 oz) can coconut milk

2 cloves garlic, crushed

1 tsp grated fresh ginger root

1/4 tsp salt

1/4 tsp black pepper

Directions

1. Wash shrimp, but don't shell them.

2. Add all ingredients to a saucepan and mix well. Bring mixture to a boil, stirring frequently.

3. When mixture starts to boil, reduce heat and simmer uncovered, stirring frequently, until shrimp are pink and firm. Serve warm.

Thai Coconut Shrimp Soup

This sweet, spicy, exotic soup is absolutely bursting with flavor!

Ingredients

1 lb medium shrimp, peeled and de-veined
3½ cups coconut milk
3 cups chicken broth
¾ cup mushrooms, sliced
¼ cup chopped fresh cilantro
3 cloves garlic, minced
1½ Tbsp grated fresh ginger
1½ tsp red chili paste
1 stalk lemongrass, chopped
3 Tbsp fish sauce
1 Tbsp honey

Salt to taste

Fresh lime wedges (for juice and garnish)

Cooking oil

Directions

1. Heat a large saucepan over medium heat and coat with oil. Add garlic, ginger, chili paste, mushrooms, and lemongrass and cook for about 3 minutes.

2. Add chicken broth, fish sauce, honey, and coconut milk to pan and stir. Bring mixture to a simmer and cook for another 15 minutes.

3. Add shrimp and cook for about 5 minutes until shrimp is cooked through.

4. To serve, transfer soup to bowls, sprinkle with salt and fresh cilantro, and squeeze on fresh lime juice.

Chipotle Lime Salmon

This recipe will satisfy your craving for something a little bit spicy. Adjust the amount of chipotle as desired.

Ingredients

1 lb salmon fillets (ideally in two fillets)

2 limes, halved

1-2 Tbsp olive oil

1 tsp chipotle powder

Salt and pepper to taste

Directions

1. Preheat oven to 425 F.

2. Rinse salmon, pat dry, and place on a metal baking sheet.

3. Rub each fillet with olive oil, and squeeze the juice from two lime halves onto each fillet (i.e. one half-lime per fillet).

4. Sprinkle fillet with chipotle powder and salt and pepper to taste, then place the remaining half-limes on top of each fillet (one half per fillet).

5. Cook fillets for 4-6 minutes per inch thickness of fillet (measuring at the fillet's thickest point. Most fillets are around 1½ inches thick, so 8-12 minutes is an approximate average. Salmon is done cooking when it flakes easily. Serve warm.

Notes

- If weather permits, this recipe is also great for grilling!

Salmon in Coconut Cream Sauce

Ingredients

1 lb salmon fillet

1 (13 oz) can coconut milk

Zest and juice of 2 lemons

3 Tbsp chopped fresh basil

6 cloves garlic, minced

2 large shallots, diced

Salt and pepper to taste

Cooking oil (coconut oil works well)

Directions

1. Preheat oven to 350 F.

2. Place salmon in a baking dish and sprinkle both sides with salt and pepper to taste.

3. Heat a sauce pan over medium heat and coat with oil. Add garlic and shallots, and saute until garlic and shallots soften, about 3-5 minutes.

4. Add lemon zest, lemon juice, and coconut milk, and bring liquid to a low boil.

5. Once mixture begins to boil, remove from heat, add basil, and stir. Pour mixture over salmon and bake uncovered for about 10-20 minutes, or until salmon has reached desired temperature. Salmon is done cooking when it flakes easily. Serve warm.

Paleo Buffalo Chicken Wraps

Lettuce wraps are one of my favorite ways to take whatever random protein I have in the refrigerator and turn it into something delicious and handheld. The crunch and freshness of lettuce wrapped around this spicy chicken is a fun change of pace from Buffalo wings.

Ingredients

1 lb boneless, skinless chicken breasts or thighs, but into 1-inch chunks
2 tsp chipotle powder
½ tsp garlic powder
½ tsp onion powder
Salt and pepper to taste

Cooking oil

(optional) hot sauce to taste

4-6 large romaine lettuce leaves
1 avocado, sliced

1 large tomato, sliced
2 Tbsp diced green onions

Directions

1. In a large bowl, toss the chicken pieces with the spices (and hot sauce, if using) until evenly coated.

2. Heat a frying pan over medium heat and coat with oil. Add chicken mixture and cook, turning occasionally, until chicken pieces are cooked through (about 5-8 minutes).

3. Spoon cooked chicken mixture into lettuce leaves, dividing evenly, and top with sliced avocado, tomato, and green onions as desired. Fold lettuce leaves into tight wraps and serve.

Cilantro Turkey Burgers

Ingredients

1 lb ground turkey

1 cup cilantro, chopped

1/4 cup red onion, chopped

2 cloves garlic, crushed

Salt and pepper to taste (1 tsp salt and ½ tsp black pepper works well)

Cooking oil (if pan frying)

Directions

1. In a bowl, combine all ingredients and mix well. Shape mixture into patties of desired size (four ¼ lb patties or two ½ lb patties work well).

2. Grill or pan fry to desired level of doneness. If pan frying, heat a frying pan over medium-high heat, coat with oil, and cook each side until browned, about 2-3 minutes per side.

Notes

- Ground turkey can be substituted for ground chicken if desired without changing the flavor of the dish too drastically.

- Although these burgers taste great on their own, they pair well with guacamole and (if you want them spicy) hot sauce!

Turkey Veggie Meatballs

Ingredients

1 lb ground turkey

2 medium carrots, peeled and roughly chopped

1 red or green bell pepper, seeded and roughly chopped

½ yellow onion, peeled and roughly chopped

½ cup fresh parsley

5 large white button mushrooms

1 clove garlic, peeled

2 Tbsp Italian seasoning (store-bought, or see Notes section to make your own)

Salt and pepper to taste (about 1 tsp of each works well)

Directions

1. Preheat oven to 350 F.

2. In a food processor, combine all ingredients except turkey and blend until veggies are finely chopped and mixture is well combined.

3. Transfer mixture to a large bowl, add ground turkey, and mix well.

4. Form mixture into meatballs of desired size (1½-2 inches in diameter works well) and transfer to a baking pan or sheet. Bake for about 25 minutes, until meatballs are cooked through. Serve warm.

Notes

- Ground turkey can be substituted for ground chicken if desired without changing the flavor of the dish too drastically.

- Italian seasoning blends can be easily and cheaply purchased at any grocery store. However, if you'd like to make your own, simply combine equal amounts of basil, thyme, oregano, marjoram, and rosemary, and mix well. If desired, you can also add an equal amount of red pepper flakes for little extra kick!

Sesame Tuna Salad

Ingredients

½ lb tuna steak or steaks, sliced into small pieces

1 cup lettuce, chopped

½ cup sesame seeds

¼ cup fresh coriander leaves, chopped

½ cup tomatoes, halved

Cooking oil (olive oil works well)

Directions

1. Spread sesame seeds evenly on a plate, then roll tuna steak/s in sesame seeds until tuna is evenly coated in seeds.

2. Heat a frying pan over medium heat and coat with cooking oil. Add tuna and cook for 1-3 minutes per side (depending on thickness of tuna pieces) until cooked through.

3. In a bowl, combine lettuce, coriander, and tomatoes and mix well. Top with tuna and serve, drizzling with olive oil (or preferred dressing) if desired.

Dilled Spinach Salad with Avocado

Ingredients

1 large handfuls baby spinach leaves

1 small beet, peeled and cut into large matchsticks

1 small avocado, peeled and chopped

¼ cup diced red onion

2 Tbsp olive oil

1 Tbsp balsamic vinegar

1 Tbsp chopped fresh dill

1-2 cloves garlic, crushed

Directions

1. In a small bowl, combine olive oil, vinegar, crushed garlic, and dill and mix well to make the dressing.

2. In a salad bowl, combine spinach, avocado, beet, and red onion and mix well. Drizzle with dressing and serve.

Salmon Burgers

Ingredients

2 cans salmon, drained

¼ cup coconut flour

3 large eggs

4 green onions, chopped

2 cloves garlic, crushed

2 Tbsp lemon juice

1 Tbsp chopped fresh dill

1 tsp mustard

¼ tsp salt

¼ tsp black pepper

Cooking oil

Directions

1. In a large bowl, whisk the eggs, then add the spices and whisk until well combined.

2. Add salmon, green onions, garlic, and dill to the bowl and mix well.

3. Add coconut flour and mix thoroughly by hand until mixture is evenly combined. Form into patties, about ½ cup of mixture per patty.

4. Heat cooking oil in a frying pan over medium-high heat. Cook patties about 4 minutes per side until golden brown.

Notes

- For a smoother texture, ingredients can be mixed prior to cooking by pulsing in a food processor until well combined.

- These burgers work well with a range of different toppings; for two tasty places to start, try guacamole and mango salsa!

Low Carb Paleo Side Dishes

Since a low-carb diet tends to be more restricted than a higher-carb diet, when you cut your carb intake you run the risk of also accidentally losing vital micronutrients that are important for good health.

The most common way this manifests itself on a low-carb paleo diet is with the reduction or elimination of fruit and starchy vegetables like sweet potatoes, as well as some nuts and other miscellaneous foods. Losing these sources of nutrition makes it necessary to make those nutrients up from other, lower-carb sources, mainly veggies.

These side dish recipes are designed to give you the best of both world's: adding healthy, nutrient-rich, low-carb vegetables to your diet, in a way that doesn't make you feel like your parents are forcing you to eat your veggies before you can go outside and play!

We think you'll find these dishes not only extremely healthy and nourishing, but also flavorful, tasty, and fun to eat. Enjoy!

Tangy Red Cabbage Slaw

Ingredients

½ head red cabbage, shredded

1 large carrot, peeled and shredded

2 scallions, chopped

½ cup Paleo Mayonnaise (see recipe in this book)

2-3 tsp sesame seeds (preferably white)

1 tsp grated fresh ginger root

Juice of ½ lemon

(optional) ¼ cup mandarin oranges or diced pineapple

Directions

1. In a bowl, combine all ingredients except fruit (if using) and sesame seeds and mix well, until veggies are thoroughly coated.

2. Mix in fruit (if using) and sprinkle with sesame seeds. Serve at room temperature or chilled.

Notes

- If you like your veggies extra crispy, you can serve this immediately after making it. Otherwise, if you make it the day before and allow it to sit overnight (anywhere up to 24 hours), the lemon juice in the mixture will tenderize the tough cabbage leaves and make the dish a bit softer. This also allows the flavors to "meld" overnight.

Low-Carb Paleo Rice (aka Cauliflower Rice)

Cauliflower is a healthy vegetable that is both low carb and high in beneficial nutrients. It's also mild-tasting, and when prepared properly has soft grainy texture that allows it to very closely mimic boiled white rice. The only difference is that it's light and healthy, and won't weigh you down like a ton of bricks after eating it!

This basic recipe is completely unflavored, just like actual boiled white rice – once you've learned how to make it, you can flavor it however you'd like, or combine it with whatever sauces, condiments, meat dishes, and other foods you'd normally pair rice with. It goes particularly well with Asian-themed dishes, as you might expect, but the possibilities are endless.

Ingredients
1 head cauliflower
1 Tbsp water

Directions

1. Cut leaves from cauliflower by slicing through the stem between the head and leaves with a knife; remove and discard leaves and stem. Cut around core with knife, being careful not to separate florets from head. Remove and discard core, then rinse florets to clean.

2. Pour 1 inch of water into a large saucepan. Place cauliflower in water, stem side down and cover. Bring to a boil over high heat, then reduce heat to low and simmer 10 to 12 minutes until cauliflower is tender. Drain and allow to cool.

3. Break florets apart and place in a food processor. Process carefully (in short pulses if necessary) until cauliflower has been evenly chopped to the consistency of rice (be

careful not to over-process it, or it will get pulverized into mush). Remove from food processor, drain off any excess liquid that has accumulated, and serve warm.

Notes

- For expediency, you can usually find bags of frozen cauliflower florets at most grocery stores that can simply be cooked in the microwave. These cooked florets can then be processed to a rice-like consistency as normal.

Low-Carb Paleo Mashed Potatoes (aka Cauliflower Mash)

Another creative and tasty use for cauliflower, this recipe is super low-carb, nutritious, extremely easy to make, and is a perfect substitute for normal, starchy, non-paleo mashed potatoes. Be sure to check the Notes section for tasty variations on the basic recipe.

Ingredients (basic recipe)

1 head fresh cauliflower, or 1 package frozen cauliflower
4 Tbsp butter

Salt and pepper to taste

Directions

1. If using frozen cauliflower, simply microwave until hot. If using fresh cauliflower, steam for 15-20 minutes until soft.

2. Transfer cauliflower to a food processor and pulse until lightly chopped. Add butter, and process until mixture is thoroughly combined and takes on a smooth consistency. Transfer to bowls, season with salt and pepper to taste, and serve warm.

Notes

- Here are a few handy variations you can use to dress this simple dish up quite a bit:

    - For garlic mashed potatoes, add 1-3 cloves crushed garlic before processing (depending on how strong you want the garlic taste to be!).

    - Add diced bacon pieces to the final dish; this works particularly well with garlic mashed potatoes. You can also incorporate the leftover bacon fat from the frying pan into the mash before processing.

    - Try sprinkling with fresh chives, or adding in finely sliced green onion.

    - Using ¼ cup or so of chicken broth instead of the butter makes the dish a bit less creamy but adds a rich, subtle flavor that you may prefer.

Sauteed Brussels Sprouts with Shallots and Pecans

Although Brussels sprouts aren't normally on anyone's list of favorite foods, they actually taste wonderful when prepared with a good recipe. This one will help you transform the much-maligned Brussels sprout into a nutrient-rich and flavorful side dish.

Ingredients

½ lb Brussels sprouts, de-stemmed and cut lengthwise into 1/4-inch thick slices

1 handful pecans (ideally raw), roughly chopped

2 small shallots, chopped

Walnut oil to taste

Cooking oil (olive oil works well

Directions

1. Heat a frying pan over medium heat and coat with cooking oil. Add the Brussels sprouts, pecans, and shallots and cook, stirring frequently, until the Brussels sprouts are tender and slightly browned (typically about 7-8 minutes). While cooking, continue to coat mixture with oil if necessary to prevent scorching.

2. When ready to serve, drizzle with walnut oil and toss. Serve warm.

Southern-Style Collard Greens

Collard greens aren't a commonly used vegetable in most parts of the country, but this classic southern recipe is a perfect showcase for this flavorful and highly nutritious plant.

Ingredients

2 bunches collard greens, de-stemmed and roughly chopped
½-1 lb bacon
1 medium yellow or white onion, diced
3 cloves garlic, crushed
1 tsp black pepper

Directions

1. Heat a large stock pot over medium heat and add bacon. Cook until crispy, then remove from pot and set aside, leaving the melted bacon fat in the pot.

2. Add garlic and onions to pot and saute in bacon at until onions are translucent.

3. Add collard greens to pot and stir until coated in bacon fat and well-mixed with the garlic and onion. Cook, stirring frequently, until they've wilted to about half their original size.

4. Sprinkle mixture with black pepper, then pour in enough water to completely cover greens. Stir well and bring to a slight boil. Reduce heat and let simmer for 30–40 minutes, until greens become tender.

5. Chop cooked bacon into rough chunks of desired size. Remove collard greens from pot and place in large serving bowl. Garnish with chopped bacon, and serve warm.

Notes

- Although this recipe is probably best with collard greens, it also works well with other tough greens, like mustard greens and kale, if you ever want to try changing things up.

- If the pot you're using isn't very big, you can add the greens to it slowly, one handful at a time, during step 3. The greens will naturally wilt and reduce in size as they cook. This allows you to use a smaller stock pot, a large saucepan, etc.

- If you like spicy food, this dish is great with hot sauce.

Rosemary Pecan Green Beans

Ingredients

1 lb. fresh green beans, trimmed

2 green onions, sliced

1 Tbsp chopped fresh rosemary

¼ cup chopped pecans

1-2 tsp lemon juice

½ tsp salt

Cooking oil (olive oil works well)

Directions

1. Sprinkle green beans evenly with ¼ tsp salt and place in a steamer basket over boiling water. Cover and steam 10 minutes or until crisp-tender. Remove from heat, drain, and set aside.

2. Heat a frying pan over medium-high heat and coat with oil. Add green onions and rosemary and saute for 2-3 minutes until softened.

3. Add green beans, pecans, lemon juice, and remaining ¼ tsp salt and stir until mixture is warmed evenly. Garnish with fresh rosemary sprigs if desired, and serve warm.

Notes

- Frozen green beans can easily be substituted for fresh ones if convenient, and the pecans can be replaced with other nuts fairly easily as well (although softer nuts, like pecans and walnuts, tend to go well with the tender cooked green beans).

Jicama Fries (i.e. Low-Carb Paleo French Fries)

If going paleo causes you to miss starchy, potato-based comfort foods like french fries, this recipe is for you. Jicama is a healthy root vegetable that, among other things, makes for a great french fry replacement that is healthy, low-carb, and paleo approved!

Ingredients

1 Jicama (about 1 lb), peeled and cut into ¼-inch thick fries

1 Tbsp olive oil

(optional) 1 tsp paprika

(optional) ½ tsp onion powder

(optional) ½ tsp garlic powder

Salt and pepper to taste

Directions

1. Preheat oven to 400 F, and place a cooling/cake rack onto a sheet pan.

2. Place the jicama in a microwave-safe bowl with 1-2 Tbsp water. Cover bowl and microwave for 6 minutes (this will prevent the jicama from staying too crisp and raw inside when the outside bakes).

3. Drain jicama of any remaining water and transfer to a dry bowl. Toss with olive oil until fries are uniformly covered in oil. Continue to toss while gradually sprinkling with salt and pepper to taste, as well as any spices you may be using, until fries are evenly coated with seasoning.

4. Spread fries evenly on cooling rack and place pan in oven. Bake for 25-30 minutes, until crispy. Serve warm.

Notes

- These fries don't go as well with ketchup as regular potato-based fries (since jicama isn't quite as starchy as potato), but they work really well with creamy sauces like ranch (as long as you can make a dairy-free, paleo-friendly version), and are amazing with guacamole!

- To spice these fries up a little, try adding cayenne pepper to your seasoning mix (adjusted based on how spicy you'd like them: start experimenting with ¼ tsp and work your way up from there).

- Although baking these fries makes them feel and taste more like regular french fries, jicama (unlike potato) can be eaten raw if you prefer (either for convenience, or because you happen to prefer the taste and texture of raw jicama). For raw fries, simply omit steps 2 and 4 (i.e. simply toss the raw jicama fries with olive oil and seasoning), and serve at room temperature.

Simple Kale Chips

A great alternative to the carb-heavy, industrial-oil-fried potato chips found in grocery stores, made from kale, one of the most nutrient-rich vegetables around. Although fairly different in taste and texture from potato chips, these work well with many of the same dips and condiments you would normally use potato chips for, especially rich, fatty foods like guacamole!

Ingredients

1 bunch kale
1 Tbsp melted oil or fat (coconut oil and bacon fat work well)
Salt and pepper to taste

(optional) 1/2-1 tsp garlic powder

Directions

1. Preheat oven to 350 F.

2. Rinse the kale leaves under cold water, pat them dry with a towel, then cut the leaves off of the stalk.

3. Cut the kale leaves into large pieces, and place them in a large mixing bowl. Top the kale with your melted fat/oil of choice, and massage the oil gently into the kale, spreading it evenly over all of the leaves.

4. Arrange the kale in a single layer on two baking sheets, and sprinkle them with garlic powder (if using), salt, and pepper to taste. Bake for 10-15 minutes or until the kale becomes crispy

Notes

- Keep a close watch on the kale as it bakes: the leaves are relatively thin and delicate, so they'll burn easily if you aren't careful!

- You can easily season these chips with any spices you want, and customize the flavor to whatever you're dipping. For a Mexican flavor you can use a taco seasoning blend, to make it spicy you can add cayenne pepper, etc.

Paleo Mayonnaise

Ingredients

1 cup light tasting olive oil (try a brand that makes "extra light olive oil", like Bertolli or Filippo Berio)

1 egg (large or extra large)

1 Tbsp vinegar (white wine and apple cider vinegar both work well, but any will do)

1 tsp mustard

1 tsp salt

Directions

1. Add egg, mustard, and vinegar to a blender and blend on low until well combine (just a few seconds).

2. Leave blender running on low, and begin to very slow dribble the olive oil into the blender, one drop at a time. Be cautious, and literally add the olive oil drop by drop at first, allowing the drops to blend thoroughly. The mixture will slowly begin to thicken as you do this; this is called "emulsification", which just means you're mixing two liquids that are normally un-mixable.

3. Once the mixture begins to thicken, you can start to add the olive oil a bit more quickly; about a teaspoon at a time. Just continue taking it slowly, and allowing each dollop of olive oil to blend thoroughly before adding the next one.

4. Continue adding more and more olive oil until it has all been incorporated into the mixture. When the mayonnaise has thickened to your desired consistency, add salt and blend another few seconds to mix. Remove from blender, transfer to an airtight container, and store in refrigerator.

Notes

- Mayonnaise pairs very well with herbs and spices: you can try spicing it up with cayenne pepper or hot sauce, adding flavorful herbs like basil or cilantro, etc. Generally speaking, these ingredients should simply be stirred into the mayonnaise after the blending/emulsifying process is complete.

- Olive oil is a great base for mayonnaise because it's mild-tasting, inexpensive, and readily available. However, you can use any mixture of healthy oils you prefer. For example, a mixture of half olive oil and half coconut oil works well. Walnut oil, avocado oil, and macadamia nut oil also work well (either partially or fully replacing the olive oil). You can even use bacon fat if you want to make "baconnaise".

- For best results, all ingredients should be at room temperature when preparing this recipe. Although not strictly necessary, it really does make a difference, and your final product will turn out creamier as a result.

- Using light-tasting olive oil (like "extra light olive oil") is also highly recommended. If you use extra virgin olive oil, the olive oil flavor will probably be too strong.

Basic Salsa

Ingredients

6 tomatoes, quartered or roughly chopped
1/2 bunch cilantro
1/2 of a white onion, peeled and quartered or roughly chopped
juice of 1 lime

1 Tbsp olive oil
1-3 cloves garlic, peeled

1-2 jalapeño peppers
Salt and pepper to taste

Directions

1. Add all ingredients to a food processor and pulse carefully until desired consistency is reached. Alternately, chop all ingredients by hand to desired consistency, drizzle with olive oil and lime juice, and mix well.

Low Carb Paleo Desserts

Obviously, one of the main things people miss when reducing their carb intake are their favorite sugary desserts. For weight loss purposes, many paleo dieters find it necessary to reduce or eliminate even relatively healthy foods from their diet if those foods contain high amounts of carbohydrates (honey, sweet potatoes, etc). This can lead to a strong craving for sweet foods in many individuals, which can be one of the biggest obstacles to maintaining a successful low-carb diet!

All the dessert recipes in this section have been designed specifically to get around this problem. Each recipe is sweetened with either moderate-carb foods like fruit, or zero-carb, paleo-friendly artificial sweeteners, giving them few or no carbs. You'll find options here that will fit any type of low-carb diet, no matter how strict, and we think you'll find all of these options will satisfy even the strongest sweet tooth in a way that is healthy, paleo-friendly, and delicious!

Note: for a discussion of paleo-friendly artificial sweeteners, including advice on adjusting the sweetness of a dish, finding the right brand of sweetener for your taste buds, and more, please see the section on artificial sweeteners in the "Ingredient Discussion" chapter.

Homemade Hot Cocoa

Ingredients

4 packets stevia

1 cup unsweetened almond milk

1-1½ Tbsp unsweetened cocoa powder

(optional) cinnamon to taste (about ¼ tsp is a good place to start experimenting)

(optional) vanilla to taste (about ½ tsp is a good place to start experimenting)

Directions

1. In a small bowl, combine stevia, cocoa powder, and cinnamon (if using) and mix well.

2. Heat a saucepan over medium heat and add almond milk and vanilla (if using). While milk heats, gradually whisk in cocoa mixture to avoid clumping.

3. When mixture has reached desired temperature, pour into a mug, sprinkle with cinnamon if desired, and serve hot.

Notes

- For a quick-and-dirty version of this recipe, it's perfectly acceptable to warm up your almond milk in the microwave.

- If you're having issues with the cocoa powder clumping up when you add it to the almond milk, (especially if you're using a quick and dirty microwaved version of this recipe), you can easiliy obtain a smooth texture by adding the mixture to a blender and blending on low. And if you like frothy drinks, blending on higher speeds creates a nice froth.

- If you'd like to try jazzing this recipe up a bit, try adding some cayenne pepper to give the cocoa a spicy kick!

Spiced Apples

Ingredients

2 large apples (any variety), cored and sliced

2 Tbsp lemon juice

2 Tbsp butter

¼ tsp clove powder

¼ tsp ginger

¼ tsp allspice

½ tsp cinnamon

Directions

1. In a bowl, combine lemon juice and spices and mix well. Add apple slices and toss until all slices are thoroughly coated.

2. Heat a frying pan over medium heat and add butter. Remove apple slices from liquid (retaining liquid)

Place apple slices in a medium bowl. Combine remaining ingredients in a small jar and pour over apple slices. Toss gently to ensure even coating.

Notes

- Instead of retaining the liquid in Step 2 and then drizzling it over the finished apples, if you'd like you can cook the excess liquid with the apples, stirring frequently, and cooking until the liquid has reduced and thickened, and coats the apples in a light, lemon-spice syrup.

- You can regularly change the flavor of this recipe by uses different varieties of apples. This can also be used to personalize the dish to your tastes: for example, Golden Delicious apples are sweet and mild, Granny Smith's are tart, etc.

Chocolate Coconut Cookie Lumps

Ingredients

1 cup shredded coconut
2 eggs
2 Tbsp butter, melted and cooled
2 Tbsp unsweetened cocoa powder
1 pinch baking soda
½ tsp vanilla extract

¼ tsp stevia powder
Optional flavor ingredients (see notes)

Directions

1. Preheat oven to 350 F.

2. In a bowl, whisk the eggs, then add the melted butter and vanilla and mix well.

3. Add the cocoa powder, baking soda, and shredded coconut and mix until well combined (and if adding any extra ingredients for flavor, fold them in now).

4. Line a cookie sheet with parchment paper, divide batter into dollops of desired size on sheet (aiming for about 10-12 dollops works well), and flatten them with a fork. Bake for 20-30 minutes, or until cookie lumps are slightly firm to the touch. Serve warm, or at room temperature.

Notes

- If you're willing to add a small amount of extra carbs to this recipe, you can add even more flavor by incorporating fresh berries (raspberries work well), sliced or chopped nuts (like sliced almonds or chopped walnuts), or low-sugar dark chocolate chips.

Pumpkin Pie Custard

Ingredients

1 cup canned pumpkin puree

2 eggs

1 cup coconut milk

1 tsp cinnamon

1 tsp vanilla

1 tsp stevia powder

¼ tsp ginger powder

¼ tsp nutmeg

Directions:

1. Preheat the oven to 350 F.

2. In a large bowl, whisk eggs, then stir in vanilla and coconut milk and mix well. Add remaining ingredients and mix until well combined.

3. Pour the custard mixture into 6 ½-cup ramekins. Place the ramekins in a high-walled baking dish, and add enough hot water to the dish to come about halfway up the side of the ramekins (being careful not to splash any water into the custard in the ramekins).

4. Carefully place dish in oven and bake for about 40 minutes, or until a knife inserted into the center of the custard comes out clean. Serve warm, or store in the refrigerator and serve chilled!

Paleo Mocha Brownies

Who needs flour when you can use cocoa, eggs, and butter to make brownies? Okay, it's a few more ingredients than that, but these are a very simple way to make a rich and delicious treat without the grains!

Ingredients

4 oz dark chocolate, melted and cooled
½ cup unsweetened cocoa powder
¼ cup butter, melted and cooled

¼ cup coconut oil, melted and cooled
3 eggs
2 Tbsp very strongly brewed coffee
2 Tbsp finely ground coffee (as finely ground as possible)

1-2 Tbsp stevia powder

Directions

1. Preheat oven to 375 F.

2. In a bowl, whisk the eggs, then add the melted dark chocolate, butter, and coconut oil and mix well.

3. Sprinkle cocoa powder gradually into mixture while whisking steadily to avoid clumping. When cocoa powder is incorporated, add brewed coffee and coffee grounds and mix one last time until mixture is well combined.

4. Line a square baking pan with parchment paper and fill with the brownie batter. Bake for about 30 minutes or until a knife inserted in the center comes out completely clean. Garnish with a light dusting of cocoa powder and/or finely ground coffee, and serve warm, at room temperature, or even chilled.

Notes

*   If you ever plan on consuming these brownies at night, be sure to make them with decaf coffee!

Paleo Chocolate Mousse

This delightfully decadent chocolate mousse recipe is a low-carb variation of a recipe from our book *Paleo Desserts* – it's so tasty, you won't believe it's healthy!

Ingredients

1 avocado

1 cup coconut milk

1 tsp vanilla extract

1/2 cup cacao powder

2 tsp stevia (or to taste)

(optional) 1/2 cup pitted dates

(optional) cinnamon to taste

Directions

1. Soak the dates for at least 30 minutes until they're soft.

2. Peel and pit the avocado.

3. Place the avocado and dates in a food processor and process until smooth (don't stop until the dates are fully blended with the coconut milk and avocado, otherwise the mixture will turn out a little chunky).

4. Add the coconut milk, cocoa powder, honey, and vanilla, and process again until the mixture is smooth.

5. Serve at room temperature, or allow to set in the fridge for one hour.

Notes

- The dates add a nice touch of sweetness to this dish, without adding very many extra carbs on a per-serving basis (and are part of the "normal", non-artificially-sweetened version of this dish). However, as noted above, you can omit them if you're cutting carbs very drastically in your diet. Just be aware that this will cut the sweetness noticeably, so you should probably compensate by adding more artificial sweetener and/or more flavoring ingredients like vanilla, cinnamon, etc.

- For a creamier texture, you can substitute half or all of a medium-sized banana for the dates. This will usually create a smoother texture than the dates, however, bananas have a very distinct flavor, whereas the dates simply add natural sweetness, so your choice will depend on your preferences.

- You can also substitute more honey for the dates, if you'd like more sweetness *and* a smoother texture; just be careful that you aren't consuming more sugar than you want!

- The ratio of avocado to coconut milk will affect the thickness of the final product, as well as the dish's subtle underlying flavors, so you can experiment with changing this ratio to suit your preferences.

- Just before serving, you can add cacao nibs and/or fresh berries as a garnish.

- This healthy, decadent dessert is a sample recipe from one of our other recipe books, *Paleo Desserts*. If you're interested in learning how to make dozens of different healthy, delicious, paleo-friendly desserts, most of the recipes in *Paleo Desserts* can be modified to be very low-carb by simply using paleo-friendly artificial sweeteners instead of normal sweeteners. If you want a healthy way to indulge your sweet tooth, be sure to check it out! Click here to check out *Paleo Desserts.*

Thai-Inspired Bok Choy Chicken Salad

Recipe Makes 4 Servings.

Nutritional Breakdown Per Serving: 185 calories, 5 grams carbohydrates, 19 grams protein, 9 grams fat.

Salad Ingredients:

1 ¾ cup chopped grilled chicken

1/3 cup diced jicama

6 grilled and diced bok choy

1/3 cup chopped cilantro

2 ½ diced green onions

1 ¼ tbsp. sesame seeds

Dressing Ingredients:

3 tbsp. coconut cream

¾ tbsp. chopped fresh ginger

1 tsp. sriracha

1 tbsp. soy sauce

¾ tbsp. fish sauce

2 ½ tbsp. lime juice

1 tsp. honey

1 tbsp. sesame oil

Directions:

Begin by mixing the above salad ingredients together in a large mixing bowl. Stir well.

Next, pour all of the dressing ingredients into a food processor or a blender. Blend the ingredients until they're completely assimilated.

Pour the created dressing overtop the salad ingredients, and toss the salad until it's coated.

Allow the salad to chill in the refrigerator for one hour to allow the dressing to assimilate well with the salad ingredients.

Enjoy!

From the Garden Basil Chicken Salad

Recipe Makes 4 Servings.

Nutritional Breakdown Per Serving: 410 calories, 8 grams carbohydrates, 23 grams protein, 33 grams fat.

Ingredients:

2 large, shredded, and pre-cooked skinless chicken breasts

2 small pitted avocadoes

1/3 cup de-stemmed basil leaves

2 ½ tbsp. olive oil

¼ tsp. black pepper

¼ tsp. sea salt

Directions:

Begin by positioning the shredded chicken in your mixing bowl.

Next, add the olive oil, the avocado, the basil, the salt, and the pepper to a food processor. Pulse the ingredients until they're completely smooth.

Add this mixture over the shredded chicken and toss the chicken well to coat it completely. Season the chicken to taste, and allow it to rest in the refrigerator prior to serving.

Chinese-Based Cabbage Chicken Salad

Recipe Makes 4 Servings.

Nutritional Breakdown Per Serving: 207 calories, 13 grams carbohydrates, 19 grams protein, 8 grams fat.

Ingredients:

1 ¾ cup chopped and cooked chicken

4 cups shredded savoy cabbage

1/3 cup julienned scallions

1 cup julienned carrot

1/3 cup chopped cilantro

1/3 cup julienned radishes

1/3 cup chopped mint

Dressing Ingredients:

2 tbsp. sesame oil

2 ¼ tbsp. coconut vinegar

2 ½ tbsp. coconut aminos

1 diced chipotle pepper

juice from ½ lime

1 tsp. honey

3 minced garlic cloves

1 tsp. diced ginger

Directions:

Begin by mixing together the chopped and julienned carrots, cabbage, scallions, and radishes. Add the mint, the cilantro, and the chopped chicken, and toss the salad in a large mixing bowl. Next, position the salad to the side.

To create the vinaigrette, begin by removing the chipotle pepper seeds. Cover the pepper with water and allow it to sit for thirty minutes.

After thirty minutes, add the pepper to the food processor and pulse it for one minute before adding the other ingredients to the processor. Taste the vinaigrette and alter the spices, if you please.

Pour the dressing over the created salad, and toss the salad to coat.

Enjoy!

Mexican-Inspired Chicken Taco Salad

Recipe Makes 3 Servings.

Nutritional Breakdown Per Serving: 328 calories, 14 grams carbohydrates, 24 grams protein, 20 grams fat.

Ingredients:

2 tbsp. taco seasoning (created below)

½ pound shredded chicken

1/3 cup water

1 tbsp. olive oil

1 head shredded lettuce

1 diced tomato

1 diced red onion

1 small, pitted avocado

½ diced green pepper

Directions:

Begin by mixing together the taco seasoning, as followings.

Bring together 1 tsp. garlic powder, 4 tbsp. chili powder, 2 tsp. paprika

1 tsp. onion powder

1 tsp. oregano

¼ tsp. red pepper flakes

3 tsp. salt

Stir the ingredients before taking out the 2 tbsp. of the taco seasoning you require for this recipe. (Note that you can keep the seasoning for a later recipe, if you so choose.)

Next, heat the olive oil in the skillet. Add the chicken to the olive oil to give it a boost of flavor. Pour the water overtop, along with the taco seasoning. Allow the chicken mixture to simmer until the water completely evaporates.

Next, slice and dice all the other ingredients.

Create the salad by assembling together the vegetables, the chicken, etc. Toss the ingredients well, and enjoy!

Indian-Inspired Paleo Curry Chicken Salad

Recipe Makes 2 Servings.

Nutritional Breakdown Per Serving: 437 calories, 36 grams carbohydrates, 33 grams protein, 19 grams fat.

Ingredients:

1 pre-cooked and cooled chicken breast

3 minced garlic cloves

3 diced green onions

2 tbsp. coconut milk

3 tbsp. green curry paste

1/3 cup golden raisins

1/3 cup sundried tomatoes

1/3 cup diced almonds

salt and pepper to taste

Directions:

Begin by shredding the chicken. Place it in a mixing bowl.

Next, add the coconut milk, the onions, the garlic, and the curry paste. Stir well, making sure to coat the chicken.

Next, add the almonds, the raisins, and the sundried tomatoes. Stir well.

Add salt and pepper to taste, and enjoy the salad with greens.

Cilantro and Lime Tangy Chicken Salad

Recipe Makes 5 Servings.

Nutritional Breakdown Per Serving: 391 calories, 10 grams carbohydrates, 42 grams protein, 20 grams fat.

Ingredients:

3 chopped, pre-cooked chicken breasts

1 chopped cabbage

1 sliced cucumber

2 diced avocadoes

juice from 2 limes

6 minced scallions

1 cup chopped cilantro

salt and pepper to taste

Directions:

Begin by mixing together all the above ingredients in a large mixing bowl. Enjoy!

Brussels Sprouts-Based Chicken Salad

Recipe Makes 4 Servings.

Nutritional Breakdown Per Serving: 392 calories, 18 grams carbohydrates, 45 grams protein, 15 grams fat.

Ingredients:

2 chopped pre-cooked chicken breasts

2 cups Brussels sprouts

½ green apple

½ cup diced almonds

½ cup chopped grapes

1 diced white onion

Dressing Ingredients:

1 tbsp. brown mustard

2 tbsp. apple cider vinegar

1 tbsp. honey

1 ½ tbsp. olive oil

½ tsp. sea salt

½ tsp. black pepper

Directions:

Begin by slicing the Brussels sprouts in half. Do this, once more, with the green apple before slicing it into smaller pieces, like matchsticks.

Slice up the grapes, as well, along with the almonds, and the onion.

Chop the chicken, and bring all the ingredients together in a large mixing bowl.

To the side, bring all the dressing ingredients together in a small mixing bowl. Stir the ingredients until they're smooth. Pour this mixture over the Brussels sprouts, and toss the salad well.

Enjoy!

Avocado-Based Paleo Chicken Salad

Recipe Makes 5 Servings.

Nutritional Breakdown Per Serving: 336 calories, 3 grams carbohydrates, 48 grams protein, 12 grams fat.

Ingredients:

3 skinless and boneless chicken breasts, pre-cooked and shredded

1/3 diced onion

1 diced avocado

2 tbsp. lime juice

3 tbsp. cilantro

salt and pepper to taste

Directions:

Bring all the above ingredients together and mix well, making sure to mash the avocado as you go.

Enjoy this very simple recipe.

Paleo Inspiration Apple and Chicken Hash Salad

Recipe Makes 4 Servings.

Nutritional Breakdown Per Serving: 380 calories, 12 grams carbohydrates, 41 grams protein, 18 grams fat.

Ingredients:

2 chicken breasts

1 diced onion

2 tbsp. chopped sage

1 chopped apple

½ tsp. allspice

4 tbsp. coconut oil

1 tbsp. maple syrup

Directions:

Begin by mixing together the sage, the apple, the coconut oil, the onion, and the allspice in a skillet. Cook the ingredients for six minutes, until the onions have turned clear. At this time, add the maple syrup.

Chop up the chicken breasts into tiny, easy-to-eat pieces. Add these to the mixture, and cook them for ten minutes. The chicken should become well done.

Serve this chicken hash with a garden vegetable, and enjoy!

Paleo Lazy Day Chicken Veggie Soup

Recipe Makes 8 Servings.

Nutritional Breakdown Per Serving: 140 calories, 12 grams carbohydrates, 13 grams protein, 5 grams fat.

Ingredients:

2 cups shredded pre-cooked chicken

1 sliced leek

1 1/3 cup diced cauliflower

1 diced bell pepper

4 diced carrots

1 diced onion

3 sliced zucchinis

1 cup diced tomatoes

3 sliced celery ribs

3 bay leaves

3 thyme sprigs

7 cups chicken stock

4 minced garlic cloves

2 tbsp. ghee

½ tsp. sea salt

½ tsp. black pepper

Directions:

Begin by melting the ghee in a large stockpot over medium-high heat.

Add the garlic, the onion, the leek, and the pre-cooked chicken and allow them to cook in the fat for approximately six minutes. The onion should be tender.

Next, administer the remaining vegetables, the thyme, the bay leaves, and the chicken broth.

Allow the mixture to boil before turning the heat to medium-low and allowing it to simmer for twenty-two minutes. Stir every few minutes.

Season the mixture with the salt and pepper. Enjoy the soup throughout the winter season!

Kale Creation Chicken Soup

Recipe Makes 8 Servings.

Nutritional Breakdown Per Serving: 215 calories, 7 grams carbohydrates, 28 grams protein, 7 grams fat.

Ingredients:

30 ounces chicken broth

5 sliced carrots

1 entire sliced and diced head of celery

1 chopped head kale

2 diced onion

2 ½ sliced chicken breasts

salt and pepper to taste

Directions:

Begin by bringing every ingredient above, except for the kale, into a large soup pot. Cook the ingredients over medium for approximately forty-five minutes. At this time, the chicken should be fully cooked.

At this time, shred the chicken while it's in the pot.

Add the kale to the soup, and serve the soup warm. Administer salt and pepper to taste. Enjoy!

Paleo Texas-Living Chicken Tortilla Soup

Recipe Makes 8 Servings.

Nutritional Breakdown Per Serving: 215 calories, 11 grams carbohydrates, 29 grams protein, 5 grams fat.

Ingredients:

2 ½ skinless, sliced chicken breasts

1 diced onion

28 ounces canned and diced tomatoes

30 ounces chicken broth

2 ¼ cups diced celery

2 ¼ cups diced carrots

1 diced jalapeno

5 minced garlic cloves

1 chopped bunch cilantro

1 tsp. chili powder

3 tbsp. tomato paste

1 tsp. cumin

2 cups water

1 tbsp. olive oil

salt and pepper to taste

Directions:

Begin by Pouring olive oil and a fourth cup of chicken broth into a large soup pot. Add the garlic, the jalapeno, the onion, the salt, and the pepper to the large soup pot over medium-high heat. Cook the mixture well, until it's soft.

Next, add the remaining ingredients to the large soup pot. After you've added everything, pour enough water into the mixture to allow the soup to reach the very top of the soup pot. Add salt and pepper as you need it.

Next, cover the soup pot and allow the soup to cook for two hours and fifteen minutes.

At this time, shred the chicken with your wooden spoon, pressing it against the side.

Top the mixture with fresh cilantro to serve, if you please, and enjoy!

Thai-Inspired Pumpkin and Chicken Soup

Recipe Makes 5 Servings.

Nutritional Breakdown Per Serving: 273 calories, 10 grams carbohydrates, 13 grams protein, 18 grams fat.

Ingredients:

15 ounces pumpkin puree

4 cups chicken broth

13 ounces coconut milk

½ tsp. sea salt

½ cup cilantro

1 ½ tsp. red curry paste

½ cup diced green onions

½ tsp. Thai fish sauce

15 ounce can of chicken breast

3 minced garlic cloves

Directions:

Begin by mixing all the above ingredients together in a large soup pot. Stir the ingredients well, and allow them to come to a boil.

When the mixture comes to a boil, reduce the heat. Allow it to simmer for twenty minutes.

After twenty minutes, utilize an immersion blender to blend the ingredients a bit, to smooth the soup and create a layered texture.

Enjoy!

Faux Chicken Noodle Soup

Recipe Makes 10 Servings.

Nutritional Breakdown Per Serving: 261 calories, 4 grams carbohydrates, 46 grams protein, 4 grams fat.

Ingredients:

3 ½ pounds chicken breast, diced

3 chopped celery stalks

4 chopped carrots

6 minced garlic cloves

1 diced onion

1 bay leaf

10 cups water

salt and pepper to taste

¼ tsp. white pepper

½ tsp. thyme

2-inch chopped noodles, made from a zucchini, julienned

Directions:

Begin by preheating the oven to 425 degrees Fahrenheit.

Next, slice up the chicken and position the chicken in a large baking dish. Add salt and pepper. Roast the chicken in the oven for twenty-five minutes.

Add the cooked chicken to a large soup pot, and add water. Bring the water to a boil on the stove over medium-high heat. Make sure to boil completely for six minutes.

Next, remove the chicken from the pot. Add the garlic, the onions, the celery, the carrots, and the bay leaf. Reduce the heat to low and allow the ingredients to simmer for forty-five minutes.

At this time, prepare the noodles from the zucchini. Add the zucchini and the chicken back to the pot, and allow the soup to simmer for six minutes.

Enjoy this fake chicken noodle soup!

Chicken Sausage Farm Days Soup

Recipe Makes 8 Servings.

Nutritional Breakdown Per Serving: 271 calories, 17 grams carbohydrates, 22 grams protein, 12 grams fat.

Ingredients:

5 sliced and peeled carrots

2 tbsp. olive oil

1 diced onion

1 ½ pound Italian chicken sausage

6 minced garlic cloves

10 ounces sliced cherry tomatoes

½ tsp. red pepper flakes

½ tsp. black pepper

8 cups chicken broth

10 ounces chopped broccoli

Directions:

Begin by slicing and dicing the onions and the garlic.

Slice the carrots.

Next, remove the chicken sausage from its casing. Trim the broccoli, and slice it up into chunks.

Heat a soup pot over medium-high heat on the stove. After three minutes, add the olive oil into the mixture, and cook the onions and the carrots, stirring every few minutes, for a full ten minutes. The carrots should be tender.

Next, add the garlic and the chicken sausage to the mixture. Cook for seven minutes, continually breaking up the chicken sausage to create chunks.

Next, remove this created mixture from the soup pot and place it to the side. Add the tomatoes to the pot, now, and cook them for four minutes. They should blister. Press each tomato to the side of the pot, at this time, making sure to burst them. Burst all of the tomatoes.

Add the chicken sausage creation back to the tomato pot. Stir well, and cook everything together for two minutes.

Next, pour the broth into the soup pot, and allow the broth to boil. When it begins to boil, add the broccoli and cook for an additional four minutes.

At this time, remove the soup from the heat. Adjust any seasonings as you please, and serve the soup warm.

Enjoy!

Paleo White Winter Wonderland Chicken Chili

Recipe Makes 6 Servings.

Nutritional Breakdown Per Serving: 328 calories, 13 grams carbohydrates, 43 grams protein, 9 grams fat.

Ingredients:

1 ¾ pound chopped chicken breasts

2 diced jalapenos

1 tbsp. olive oil

2 diced onions

1 diced green pepper

1 tsp. coriander

5 minced garlic cloves

5 cups chicken broth

4 tbsp. arrowroot powder

4 tbsp. coconut milk

5 ounces green chiles

Directions:

Begin by chopping up the chicken and the vegetables.

Position a large soup pot over medium-high heat, and cook the onions, the peppers, the oli, the jalapenos, and the garlic in the olive oil for five minutes.

After five minutes, add the salt, the spices, and the chicken. Allow the chicken to sauté for an additional seven minutes.

Pour the broth, the coconut milk, and the green chiles into the soup pot before adding the arrowroot powder slowly. Whisk well.

Allow the soup to come to a boil before lowering the heat to medium-low and allowing it to simmer for twenty-two minutes.

At this time, mash the chicken and create shreds. Serve the chili warm, and enjoy!

Delicious Chipotle Chicken Chili

Recipe Makes 8 Servings.

Nutritional Breakdown Per Serving: 202 calories, 6 grams carbohydrates, 33 grams protein, 3 grams fat.

Ingredients:

2 pounds shredded and cooked chicken

1 cup chicken stock

3 chopped onions

¾ pound chopped tomatoes

3 tbsp. apple cider vinegar

5 minced garlic cloves

3 tbsp. coconut aminos

1 tbsp. chipotle powder

1 tsp. cumin

1 tsp. paprika

1 tsp. cayenne pepper

1 tsp. oregano

1 tsp. black pepper

1 tsp. sea salt

Directions:

Begin by bringing the above ingredients into a large soup pot. Stir the ingredients well.

Allow the mixture to come to a boil before covering the pot. Reduce the heat to low and allow it to simmer for four hours.

Enjoy!

Mexican-Inspired Chicken Chili

Recipe Makes 4 Servings.

Nutritional Breakdown Per Serving: 407 calories, 24 grams carbohydrates, 45 grams protein, 14 grams fat.

Ingredients:

1 ¼ pound skinless and boneless chicken breasts

1 diced onion

4 minced bell peppers

2 ¼ cup salsa

1 diced jalapeno pepper

2 cups water

3 minced garlic cloves

1 tsp. chili powder

1 tsp. cumin

1 diced avocado

salt and pepper to taste

Directions:

Begin by bringing together the garlic, the salsa, the chicken breasts, the cumin, the water, the onion, the chili powder, the salt, and the pepper into a large soup pot. Stir well before covering the soup pot and allowing it to simmer on low for three hours.

Next, remove the chicken from the soup pot and shred it before returning it back to the soup pot.

At this time, saute the jalapeno and the bell peppers in a skillet with a bit of olive oil for five minutes. Add these to the soup pot. Stir well, and cover once more.

Allow the chili to continue to simmer for twenty-five minutes.

Add the avocado to the top of the chili prior to serving, and enjoy!

Recipe Makes 10 Servings.

Nutritional Breakdown Per Serving: 370 calories, 9 grams carbohydrates, 49 grams protein, 14 grams fat.

Ingredients:

3 ½ pound chicken

1/3 cup ghee

3 minced garlic cloves

3 diced onions

2 cups chicken broth

1/3 cup almond flour

3 diced carrots

5 sliced mushrooms

1 cup green peas, either fresh or frozen

3 sliced green onions

1/3 cup coconut milk

salt and pepper to taste

Directions:

Begin by slicing and dicing the chicken.

To the side, melt the ghee in a saucepan and add the chicken. Cook the chicken until it's browned on all sides. When it's done, place it to the side.

Next, add the onions to the saucepan. Cook the onion in the ghee. After they've begun to brown, add the garlic. Cook for an additional six minutes.

At this time, add the almond flour to the onion and the garlic, and stir well. Pour the chicken broth into the mixture. Stir well, administering more broth if you feel the stew is too thick.

Next, add the chicken and the vegetables to the stew. Season the stew with any salt and pepper.

When the stew comes to a simmer, cook the stew on low. Maintain the simmer. Cover the stew and allow it to cook for thirty-five minutes.

Next, add the coconut milk, the peas, and the green onions, and cook for an additional two minutes.

Enjoy!

Mediterranean Chicken Stew

Recipe Makes 4 Servings.

Nutritional Breakdown Per Serving: 436 calories, 13 grams carbohydrates, 62 grams protein, 14 grams fat.

Ingredients:

1 ¾ pounds chopped chicken

28 ounces chopped tomatoes

8 minced garlic cloves

30 olives

2 cups chicken broth

2 tbsp. minced basil

2 tbsp. minced rosemary

2 tbsp. minced parsley

1 tbsp. ghee

salt and pepper to taste

Directions:

Begin by preheating the oven to 325 degrees Fahrenheit.

Next, salt and pepper each piece of chicken. Melt the ghee in an oven and stovetop-safe dish, and then brown each of the chicken pieces for three minutes. Add the garlic to the dish, as well, along with the olives, the tomatoes, the rosemary, the chicken broth, and the thyme. Cover the dish and position it in the preheated oven for sixty minutes.

Net, add the parsley and the basil to the dish and position the dish back in the oven, this time without a cover, for forty minutes.

Enjoy!

African-Inspired Chicken Stew

Recipe Makes 4 Servings.

Nutritional Breakdown Per Serving: 470 calories, 15 grams carbohydrates, 47 grams protein, 24 grams fat.

Ingredients:

1 tbsp. coconut oil

1 ¼ pound skinless chicken breasts

1 diced onion

salt and pepper to taste

4 minced garlic cloves

1-inch diced piece ginger

1 bay leaf

½ tbsp. coriander

1/3 cup water

1 ¼ cup crushed tomatoes

1/3 cup sunflower butter

¼ tsp. vanilla

Directions:

Begin by salting and peppering the chicken well.

Heat a large Dutch oven over medium-high for approximately four minutes. Add the coconut oil to the bottom and allow it to melt.

Next, place the chicken at the bottom and brown the chicken on each of its sides. After the chicken browns, place it to the side.

Next, cook the ginger and the onions in the pot until they're soft. This should take about eight minutes. Next, add the coriander, the garlic, and the bay leaf. Cook for approximately one minute before adding the water and the tomatoes. Stir well.

Place the chicken inside the created sauce.

Boost the heat to high to allow it to boil. When it begins to boil, reduce the heat to medium-low and cook for twenty-five minutes, covered.

Afterwards, remove the chicken from the pot. Break it up.

Next, add the sunflower butter and the vanilla to the soup pot. Stir well. Add the chicken back to the stew and cover, allowing it to cook for an additional six minutes.

Serve the stew warm, and enjoy.

Thai-Inspired Kid-Friendly Paleo Chicken Pizza

Recipe Makes 4 Servings.

Nutritional Breakdown Per Serving: 355 calories, 32 grams carbohydrates, 17 grams protein, 19 grams fat.

Paleo Pizza Crust Ingredients:

2 ¼ cups almond flour

½ tsp. sea salt

½ tsp. garlic powder

2 eggs

½ tsp. baking soda

1 tbsp. olive oil

Pizza Ingredients:

1 minced garlic cloves

2 tbsp. apple cider vinegar

1 de-seeded red chili

1/3 cup honey

1/3 cup water

½ tsp. arrowroot starch

1 egg yolk

¾ cup shredded and pre-cooked chicken

1 diced red onion

½ diced red pepper

1/3 diced zucchini

4 tbsp. coconut milk

Directions:

Begin by preheating the oven to 425 degrees.

To the side, begin by creating the paleo pizza crust. Stir together the almond flour, the salt, the garlic powder, the eggs, the soda, and the olive oil. You can use a food processor if you want it to be really smooth. Then, spread the paleo pizza crust, and bake it for eight minutes in the preheated oven.

At this time, prepare the rest of the pizza.

Place the red chili, the vinegar, the garlic, and the salt together in a food processor, and pulse the ingredients until they're chopped.

Pour this created mixture into a saucepan, and add the arrowroot starch and just one tbsp. of the water. Add the honey, and bring the mixture to a simmer, stirring all the time.

After the mixture begins to thicken, remove it from the heat and place it to the side.

At this time, spread the created sauce overtop the pizza crust. Add the vegetables overtop the chili sauce, followed by the chicken.

Next, to the side, stir together the egg yolk and the coconut milk to the side. Pour this mixture over the toppings.

Bake the pizza for ten minutes, until the crust is golden.

Enjoy the pizza warm.

Finger Lickin' Good Kid-Friendly Chicken Wings

Recipe Makes 10 Servings.

Nutritional Breakdown Per Serving: 279 calories, 10 grams carbohydrates, 36 grams protein, 9 grams fat.

Ingredients:

2 ¾ pound separated chicken wings

1/3 cup lemon juice

1/3 cup honey

1/3 cup water

2 tbsp. tamari soy sauce

2 tsp. garlic powder

2 ½ tbsp. apple cider vinegar

1 tsp. ground ginger

Directions:

Begin by bringing the lemon juice, the honey, the soy sauce, the water, the garlic, the vinegar, and the ginger together in a saucepan. Heat it over medium-high, stirring a bit. When it begins to simmer, turn the heat to low and allow it to simmer for five minutes before allowing it to cool.

Pour this mixture over the chicken wings. Allow the chicken to marinate in the refrigerator for three hours.

Next, preheat the oven to 400 degrees Fahrenheit. Bake the chicken wings for sixty minutes in the preheated oven, making sure to turn them over after thirty minutes.

Enjoy!

Paleo Kid-Friendly Chicken Fingers

Recipe Makes 4 Servings.

Nutritional Breakdown Per Serving: 314 calories, 6 grams carbohydrates, 37 grams protein, 15 grams fat.

Ingredients:

1 pound no-bone, no-skin chicken, sliced into chicken fingers

1 cup shredded coconut

1 ¼ cup almond flour

1 tsp. paprika

1 egg

½ tsp. garlic powder

1 tsp. onion powder

½ tsp. cumin

Directions:

Begin by preheating the oven to 375 degrees Fahrenheit.

Next, lay out the chicken strips on a piece of parchment paper. Season both sides of the chicken with the paprika, the garlic, the cumin, and the onion powder.

To the side, whisk up the egg. In another bowl, stir together the coconut and the almond flour.

Dip the chicken strips first in the egg, then in the flour mixture. Coat each of them well.

Place the chicken strips on a baking sheet, and bake them for twenty minutes.

Enjoy!

Ranch-Flavored Kid-Friendly Chicken Nuggets

Recipe Makes 5 Servings.

Nutritional Breakdown Per Serving: 279 calories, 4 grams carbohydrates, 30 grams protein, 15 grams fat.

Ingredients:

1 pound boneless, skinless, bite-sized chicken pieces

½ tsp. dried dill

½ tbsp. parsley

½ tsp. onion powder

½ tsp. garlic powder

½ cup coconut milk

½ tsp. basil

1 egg

2 ¼ cup almond flour

Directions:

Begin by preheating the oven to 375 degrees Fahrenheit.

To the side, mix together the dill, the parsley, the onion powder, the garlic powder, the pepper, the basil, the egg, and the coconut milk in a small bowl. Pour this fake ranch into a large storage bag.

Add the pieces of chicken to the bag, as well, and shake the sealed bag well to coat the chicken.

Add the almond flour to the bag and continue to shake to give it a nice coating.

Position the chicken nuggets on a baking sheet and bake them for twenty minutes. They should be golden brown.

Enjoy!

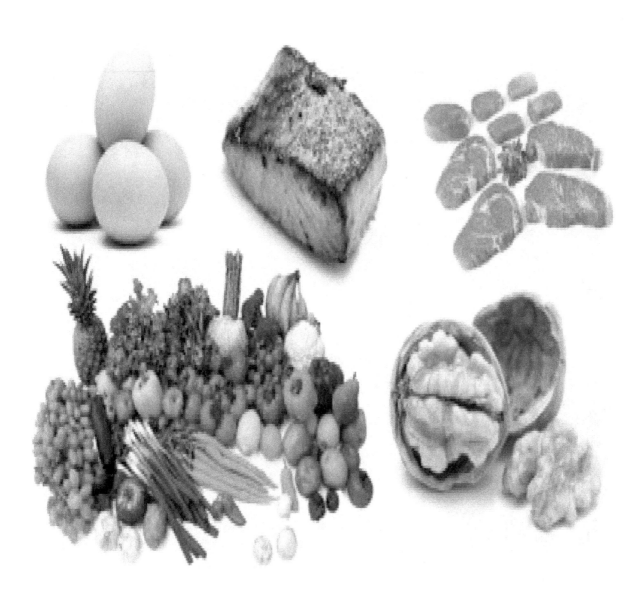

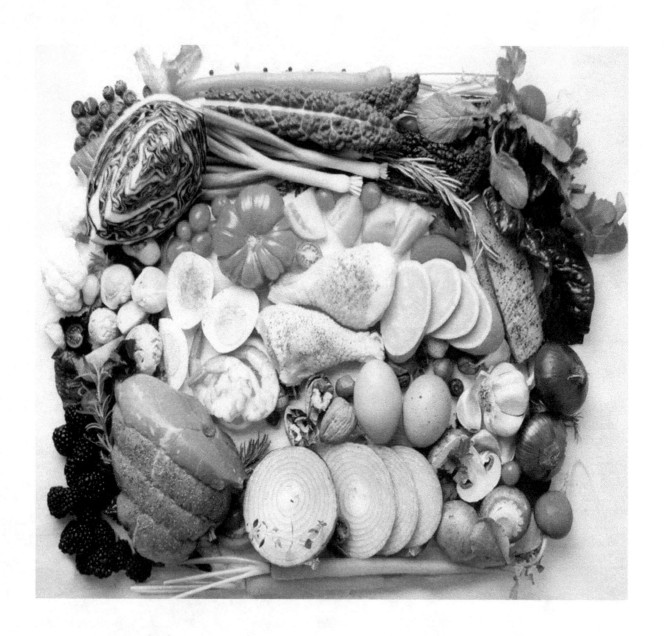

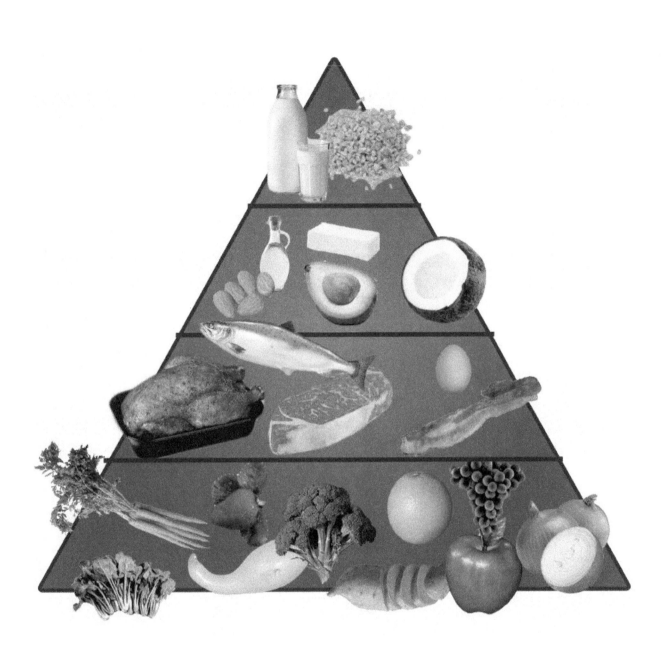

CPSIA information can be obtained
at www.ICGtesting.com
Printed in the USA
BVHW010650300721
613018BV00052B/871